Shannon -
So Good to Make
Friends with You
Look forward to
Great Years Ahead

MORE THAN A PACE HORSE

It doesn't matter what platform you started with, it only matters what platform you're standing on now

More Than a Pace Horse

It doesn't matter what platform you started with, it only matters what platform you're standing on now

Steve Qualls

XULON PRESS

Xulon Press
2301 Lucien Way #415
Maitland, FL 32751
407.339.4217
www.xulonpress.com

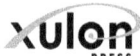

© 2019 by Steve Qualls

All rights reserved solely by the author. The author guarantees all contents are original and do not infringe upon the legal rights of any other person or work. No part of this book may be reproduced in any form without the permission of the author. The views expressed in this book are not necessarily those of the publisher.

Unless otherwise indicated, Scripture quotations taken from the English Standard Version (ESV). Copyright © 2001 by Crossway, a publishing ministry of Good News Publishers. Used by permission. All rights reserved.

Printed in the United States of America.

ISBN-13: 978-1-5456-7100-9

I dedicate this book to:

My wife Tena Qualls
My son and daughter-in-law Taylor and Sami
My daughter and son-in-law Amy and Joel
My grandchildren,
Zach, Kaylee, Ian, Bryah, Kenzi, Salem

Special thanks and recognition to
Christpoint Church
I love you all.

Thank you
Next Level Relational Network

And to you, remember,
You're more than a pace horse;
You're God's favorite

Steve Qualls is the lead pastor of Christpoint church of Tennessee. He and his wife Tena serve and lead forward in a real way. Pastor Steve refers to himself as a ditchdigger that God called out of the ditch and into the pulpit. He has pushed past the stuttering and learning disabilities he possesses and speaks in a relevant and dynamic way to break down the Word of God to real people. Their heart is to reach the lost and encourage the believer.

We pray as you read *More than a Pace Horse*, you see in yourself as more than the issues you have or the past labels you carry. You have more value than you think, and you're more important to God than you'll ever know.

For more information or speaking engagements:

www.christpoint.church
pastor@christpoint.church
fb—Steve Qualls
fb—More than a Pace Horse

Contents

Introduction ix
Chapter 1 The Beaten Horse 1
Chapter 2 The Workhorse 13
Chapter 3 The Mustang 25
Chapter 4 The Lead Horse 35
Chapter 5 The Mare 47
Chapter 6 The Stray Horse 57
Chapter 7 The Dead Horse 67
Chapter 8 The Dark Horse 77
Chapter 9 The Trojan Horse 85
Chapter 10 The Pace Horse 97
Chapter 11 The Thoroughbred 107
Chapter 12 The Stampede 119

INTRODUCTION

I graduated valedictorian, number one in my class. I was voted most likely to succeed by my peers. I finished college early with a perfect 4.0. I was fast-tracked and became a CEO of a major corporation before the age of forty.

Yeah, that's not me. I'm the dyslexic, ADD, ADHD ditchdigger from Sparta, Tennessee, who stutters when he speaks. Reading was very difficult because I possessed a learning disability that I didn't even know I had. What I did read I had difficulty processing because of my ADD. And what did slip through had a hard time staying there because of the hyper portion that is added to the attention deficit portion of a disability I didn't ask for. But the good news is that I did get a lot of whippings. On top of all that, I'm a southern kid, born and raised, which means when I talk, I sound even more uneducated and backward.

Because of the issues going on in my brain, pretty much nothing gets filtered out. Everything is going on at the same time, so a lot of times what's said is not what was intended and what comes out is a varied compilation of the original intended message. So, let's just say that a ditchdigger from the South with a learning disability, who had trouble processing thought and difficulty speaking, would never qualify to instruct, cast vision, and teach—let alone become the lead pastor of a multi-campus church. But God has a way of using even the least of these. It's taken me a lifetime to become comfortable in my own skin. It's taken years to embrace what God has called me to and "just be" in Him.

I guess I'm writing this for the kid in the seat closest to the teacher who thinks he's the dumb one in the class because he can't keep up. Maybe it's to the person who laughs when the others laugh but really doesn't understand what was just said. It could be that you're the one who clocks in every day, doing what is right and responsible, but all the while knowing there's more out there, something greater, like the alcoholic, the recovering drug addict, the once-imprisoned felon, or the average Joe or Jane. And you, maybe this is for you—yeah, you know who you are. You're the one who says church is not for me. Those folks don't want my kind of people in their church. Well you got it all backward. It's not all about church; it's about running your race. You are the one who God has his eyes on. You are the very person who, despite all of the baggage and embarrassment, Jesus died for. You are more than a pace horse; you are God's thoroughbred. We just have to get you out and let you run.

> "You are more than a pace horse; you are God's thoroughbred."

You think, *God doesn't want me, society will never accept me, and people will never respect me.* Well, take it from a dyslexic hyperactive ditchdigger with a southern drawl and confusing speech, there's only one qualifier and His name is Jesus. Come on with me and let's roll because you're worth more to Jesus than you think. You may not understand your value, but Jesus does, so welcome home.

Chapter 1

THE BEATEN HORSE

Have you ever had someone tell you that you just can't do it? I'm not talking about the obvious. Years ago I would often use a friend of mine who was a whopping ninety pounds soaking wet as an example in youth ministry. It was clear that her calling would never be a professional wrestler. That much was obvious. I'm not even talking about the coach that took you off the mound in little league because the other kid could throw strikes and you couldn't.

Many years ago when I played little league baseball, I had never played the game before in my life. I was like that new kid "Smalls" in the movie *The Sand Lot*. My dad wasn't a very patient teacher, and he worked too many long hours to teach me to play ball, so I had to learn on the fly. It's pretty embarrassing knowing you're the only kid on the field in uniform, has a team hat, and is wearing a glove but doesn't even know the basic principles of the game. On my first practice, the coach asked me what position I played, and I didn't know what that meant. Needless to say, that first year was spent more on the splinters than on the grass. I rarely saw my father at the games, although he may have been there and I didn't know. It didn't make him a terrible father; he just simply didn't want to leave the fields and his work to watch other kids that he didn't know play a game that he wasn't interested in. So when I did play, I was stuck in right field. In case you don't know what that means, most batters are right-handed and will naturally hit toward the left side of the field. In little league, unlike college and pros, it's the place you stick your weakest link. I would stand out there, dreaming for the opportunity to make my play. I could envision diving for a line drive or robbing someone of a home run at the warning track. And when the game was over and our win was celebrated at the Dairy Queen, you hoped and prayed you could accumulate a grass or dirt stain to prove you were a contributing part of the game, even if you had to rub a little dirt on you from the dugout. The dream was bigger than the game. There was always that thought of "more."

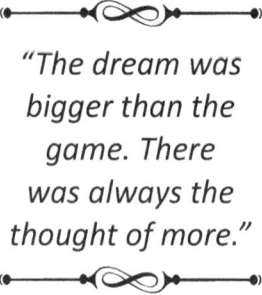

"The dream was bigger than the game. There was always the thought of more."

But something happened that changed everything in baseball for me. The coach (who I still remember to this day) asked me to play catcher. Are you kidding me! That's the coolest spot on the field. You get to wear the best gear. You're involved in every single play. You have the ability to control the game by calling the pitches, and oh yes, you can distract the opposing team's batters by talking to them. I just needed someone to believe in me—someone to give me a chance. I knew I could do it. Not only did that one position change give me confidence behind the plate as a defensive player, it also boosted my belief in myself as a hitter. I still remember the first game my dad was there to watch me play as a catcher, I went three for four that night with two doubles and a single. I was finally a baseball player! And for the first time, I felt like I was a pretty good one at that. I had earned the dirt stains and was proud of it, and it was all because a coach, who barely knew me, gave me a chance to succeed.

So the question is, has someone ever told you that you couldn't do something? Or maybe that you weren't good enough? Have they ever beaten you down and kicked you to the curb and left you for dead? Maybe their words still penetrate your very soul to this day.

In August of 1998, I sat in an office with the two greatest men in my life. One was my pastor and the other the associate pastor who was also my mentor and father in the Lord. They were my heroes. I wanted to be like them in everything I did. Their personalities were polar opposites from one another, and I was a carbon copy of my pastor, so needless to say, we were all very close. But this day was different than all the rest. This day felt cloudy from the start of the meeting, even from the first phone call. I sat in an office on a hot summer day and had a finger stuck in my face and was told, "You are a joke. You will never be able to minister. You will never become a minister. No one will ever follow anything that you teach. You are only a product of what we have made you."

My soul was sliced into pieces that day. The confidence that was built in me over the years as a successful youth pastor was shattered with a single nine-second statement. What took years to build was destroyed in a moment, much like a fire that consumes a home. I was young and unproven in warfare. This was my first major battle on the front lines, and I can say the scars are still there, though the wounds have healed. I once heard a prominent minister say that the devil fights hardest where he fears most. I must have been pretty popular to the enemy because on that day, I felt like I was his greatest fear.

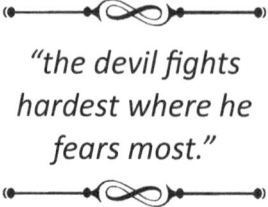

"the devil fights hardest where he fears most."

This is the classic illustration of the beaten horse. Even a horse with a spark in his eye and fierceness in his nostrils loses some of that fire when he's been beaten. My wife and I not only lost our heroes that day, we also lost our church home. All of a sudden, there was great tension, and someone had to go. The obvious choice was for Tena and me to leave the only church home we had ever known. We fought that notion for some time until God made it very clear to move. We lost our pastors, mentors, spiritual father, church, ministry, and friends in nine seconds. We felt like orphans.

Now, let me ask that question again, but I'll rephrase it a bit. Have you ever been told that you're a loser? You know most of us don't have to have a physical person tell us that, we're pretty good at self-evaluation. Our own thoughts are devastating enough to cripple us. Maybe you just need someone to believe in you. You know, give you a chance, kind of like a little league right fielder who only wants a chance to become the starting catcher.

I would like to reference two individuals from the Bible that should have been beaten down. They had every right to give up. But they didn't. Let's look at Jephthah from the Old Testament book of Judges. Chapter 11 introduces us to him as a mighty warrior. That's pretty cool if we stop right there and not read any further. I would love to be introduced as a mighty warrior, but you see there's always a nine-second response looming just around the corner, and we don't even get out of the first verse until we hear it, read it, and allow it to permeate our souls. *But*—there's that word that implies there are skeletons in the closet. *But* she's a recovering addiction. *But* he filed bankruptcy. *But* he got his girlfriend pregnant. *But* she's a woman, and women can't do that. *But* he's only a ditchdigger.

Jephthah, not to be left out, has a *but* in the middle of his story also. Verse one continues with, "*but* he was the son of a prostitute." Sometimes it doesn't matter how many people call you mighty, all you feel they remember is the *but*. All that permeates your self-esteem is that you're the son of a nobody.

> "Sometimes it doesn't matter how many people call you mighty, all you feel they remember is the but."

There are two instances I can recall that set my confidence level to an all-time high. Once when I was very young, maybe eighteen or nineteen and the other a few years later. The first happened when someone asked my father in the local coffee shop (which back then we called the diner) if he could do a small job for them with one of the pieces of equipment that he owned. Now my father was a ditchdigger. He owned a backhoe and made a living from the seat of a John Deere. He was widely sought after in our small town and had a reputation of being the best operator. When the question was asked in the diner in front of my father's peers, and even some of mine, he responded, "Just let Steve do that job for you; he is as good as I am." Of course I wasn't but that four seconds of affirmation sent my self-worth and confidence through the roof.

From that day forward, I was a different operator. (Did I mention that I was a ditchdigger?) It didn't matter what anyone really thought concerning whether I was as good as my father or not. All that matters was that he said it, and I believed it.

The other instance came from the most important person to me in this world: my wife Tena. After a few years of marriage she made a two-second statement one day to some friends that I will never forget: "That man can do anything." The power that is carried in six seconds of combined encouragement has a way of lifting the beaten horse from the side of the road and replacing the spark in the eye and putting some fierceness in his nostrils. Six seconds can be all it takes to begin to wash away nine seconds of terrorism.

Now Jephthah has way more going on than the first verse indicates. Gilead was his father, and Gilead had a wife. Now this was obviously the wife of his choosing. She's a mother and wife, not a prostitute. Gilead and his wife had other sons. Verse 2 says that she also gave him sons, and those sons grew up hating Jephthah because he had a *but* in his story. They despised him and drove him away. Just like that, Jephthah had a finger stuck in his face, and in a six-second statement, he found himself without brothers, a father, and a home. In six seconds, he was an orphan.

But here is what can happen when a beaten horse is beaten further down: everyone wants to be home whether it's pleasant or not. If we can't go home anymore, then we will make home where we are. Sometimes it's not where we need to be. Jephthah went to a place called Tob. This was a surrogate home for him. And the first thing that happened was that he drew to the worthless inhabitants of Tob.

You already feel like you're worthless yourself, with a scarred record or distorted past. Your life has a *but* in the middle. Nobody wants you. You're without friends, family, and a home. Where do most people gravitate to under these circumstances? You guessed it, the wrong crowd. These are not always the worst people; they're just the worst for you.

The word *Tob* in Hebrew means "pleasing or good." Good people can find themselves in the wrong place and around the wrong people very easily. Even mighty warriors need a home to fight for.

Although Jephthah was an outcast and rejected, there was something in there that said, "There's more." There's more than these people around me, dragging me down. There's more than being an orphan. There's more of me than I possibly think of myself.

Later on, an enemy was waging war against Jephthah's father Gilead, and the brothers came calling. They wanted Jephthah to lead them into battle against the Ammonites. He became their leader as well as their commander. Now there are some things we know about Jephthah. For starters, he was a mighty warrior with a disability he didn't ask for. We know beneath the beaten horse was a warrior looking for the coach to promote him to a better position. We do know that he is recorded in the books of Judges as a leader and judge of Israel and a catalyst for great victories. What we don't know are the nights he wept with the memory of rejection fresh in his mind. We don't know how many times he disqualified himself because he had a *but* in the middle of his story. What we don't know is how much more powerful he could have been if he had just been loved in the beginning and encouraged rather than discarded.

Now the same spirit that stuck a finger in the face of Jephthah thousands of years ago and the same spirit that stuck a finger in my face in 1998 is the same spirit that stuck a finger in our face again twenty years later. As I mentioned earlier, my wife and I pastor a wonderful church in middle Tennessee. We teamed with six people on Mother's Day 2013, and launched Christpoint Church. In our particular location in middle Tennessee, we are very rural and surrounded by other rural communities as well. Some are a bit larger than our town, and others are smaller. The city population of our town is just shy of five thousand, and our county population is just under twenty-seven thousand. We are located in the Bible Belt, and some would say the buckle. There are many churches scattered throughout our community.

I actually did a personal study as to how many churches we have compared to the number of people. Because of our smaller population and higher number of churches, we have approximately one church for every 167 people. The comparison to more populated metropolitan areas, is more like one church for several thousand people. In 2018, we launched a second campus in an even smaller neighboring community. Once again, we experienced that spirit of rejection when some of the local folks voiced their disapproval.

A finger was stuck in our face and a familiar nine-second statement was made. "You will not have a church in this town. No one will come. Good luck having a church with nobody in it." Proverbs 18:21 tells us that life and death are in the power of the tongue. With the spoken word, we possess the ability to build up or tear down. You could kind of say that we have the opportunity to beat the horse, or we can choose to restore him.

The other individual in the Bible is Jesus. Not too many things can cause the King of kings and Creator of life to marvel. After all, he knows everything all the time and at the same time. But there are two accounts recorded in scripture where Jesus marveled. One was at the great faith of a Roman centurion. The other was because of the great lack of faith from his own hometown in Mark chapter 6. Even Jesus has a *but* in his story, so you're in good company. Jesus arrives in his hometown but can't do anything because of their lack of faith.

Verse 6 shows us his ability to marvel. The very son of God himself was left amazed and astonished. He arrives on the scene, begins to speak with life changing power, and in verse 2 the energy crescendos as people are blown away by every word. The anointing builds with each sentence. Oh the wisdom and mighty works, and all of a sudden there's a *but* in verse 3. *But* isn't this just the carpenter? Isn't he the son of Mary and Joseph? This can't be the messiah, we know this guy. We know his family, played ball and fished with his brothers. Why we even know his sisters.

What started to escalate into a powerful Jesus movement was squelched with a two-second sabotage of words: "Isn't this the carpenter?" Carpenters can't be saviors. Prostitutes can't birth warriors, girls that get pregnant out of wedlock can't be used by God, alcoholics and addicts won't recover, small town churches will never grow, and ditchdiggers can't pastor churches, but don't tell that to God.

The problem with learning disabilities is the fact that you probably had it passed on to you, and you likewise pass it on to your children. We didn't have a name for it when I was in school in the seventies. Like I said, I had something wrong with me that I didn't even know I had. That is until my son came home from school one day and asked if he was dumb. We enrolled him into an after-school learning center to help him catch up. They guaranteed we would see improvement in his reading, comprehension, and overall classroom experience. We couldn't afford to pay for the classes, so the "workhorse" was called on, and we traded hours upon hours of painted murals in the facility in order to get our son the help he needed.

After the first semester they tested him and quickly informed us that he actually had regressed rather than had gotten better. They recommended us for a full study at Middle Tennessee State University. It took a year to get approved and accepted, and after two days of testing and evaluation they delivered the news: "Yep, your son is dyslexic. Now which one of you did he get it from?" I had passed this weird learning disability on to my son. To say the least, we threw parties and rewarded "C" averages. Sometimes the best we could do was a "D" minus and that was okay. But here is something I noticed in my son through the years: "He could do anything."

There was something in him that was familiar to me. His eyes would drift toward the window, his mind would wander, but in his tone you always knew he was thinking, "There's more."

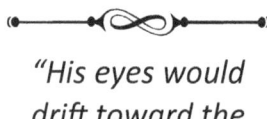

"His eyes would drift toward the window, his mind would wander, but in his tone you always knew he was thinking, "There's more.""

Once I took him and his buddies from school and church out on Halloween night to "softly terrorize" some of our friends with gifts of toilet paper. The road sign ahead on the back road told the name of the street. My son asked if that was the right road, and one of the kids in the back yelled, "What's the matter? Can't you read?" And the two nearest me laughed and said "no actually he can't."

How embarrassing that was for him that night. He was singled out and labeled with a two-second statement as the dumb kid. My heart broke for him, and I quickly changed the subject before it could get worse. His head hung a bit lower that night. A nine-year-old should never have to feel like a beaten horse. I watched him live with a *but* in his story all his life. He pulled himself away, and like Jephthah, he drew to those that made him worse. He even said once that these were the people that didn't make him feel dumb.

As soon as he turned eighteen, he began to attempt to change himself. One tattoo led to another and another until he was completely covered. Maybe this is where a therapist would say that he was trying to control the hurt or deep down inside was unhappy with himself and tried to change what he could.

Today he has a wonderful wife, marriage, and three beautiful girls, and he and his wife own their own business. There's a *but* in his story; however, it hasn't kept him from knowing *there's more*" I don't know if my words did for him what my father's words did for me, but I recently told him that he was much better at what he does than I ever was. I hope that two seconds of affirmation does for him what my father's words did for me.

What about you? What nine seconds of discouragement from the enemy is keeping you from knowing there's more? No one runs harder than the one who's told he can't keep up but is determined to show that he can. God doesn't expect you to be perfect or to even be the best. But just know that He thinks more of you than you think of yourself. Maybe you're about to clock in for your shift. You might be the one who is sitting on the sidelines, wishing you had your opportunity to play. Or, you may just be the dyslexic kid struggling to stay focused, eyes drifting toward the window, and thinking *There's more*.

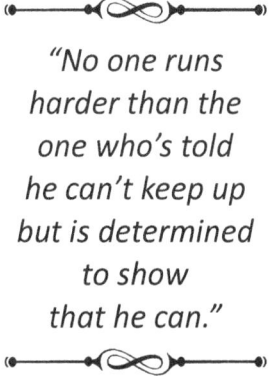

"No one runs harder than the one who's told he can't keep up but is determined to show that he can."

Chapter 2
THE WORKHORSE

There are two different types of workhorses. One is the actual workhorse himself, and the other is the packhorse. Their roles are similar but vary a bit between the two. In this chapter, let's take a look at these two types of horses and see if we can identify with either. Remember the title of the book is *More Than a Pace Horse*. As we move through the chapters, hopefully we can unearth some truths in our own lives. Maybe you have felt your role has been overlooked and your worth underappreciated along the way. This is the workhorse mentality.

Throughout these chapters, you will notice a lot of my story intertwined with biblical truths and teaching. Please note that I don't use these instances to draw attention to myself or to garner sympathy. It's what God has laid on my heart.

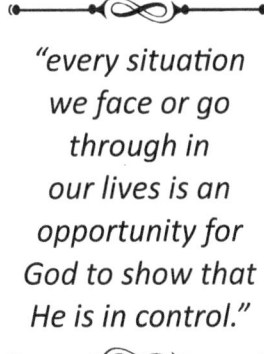

"every situation we face or go through in our lives is an opportunity for God to show that He is in control."

Each and every situation we face or go through in our lives is an opportunity for God to show that He is in control. The scripture in Romans 8:28 jumped off the page for me many years ago when I noticed that not only do things work together where God is present, He also is in full control of our lives if we truly love him. Every day is another block of time, giving Him the opportunity to show up.

As I mentioned earlier, God called me out of the ditch to minister his great gospel. But when you're a ditchdigger, you're no stranger to work. I grew up as the workhorse. My mother and father were stationed in Biloxi, Mississippi, and remained there after his discharge from the Air Force. They had decided to put down roots on the edge of the Gulf of Mexico. My father had grown up extremely poor on a farm in Tennessee. My mother grew up equally poor, pretty much living as an orphan. She was tossed about from relative to relative, separated from her siblings for many years of their lives. She once told me they had been apart for so long and from such a young age that when they did reconnect, they didn't know one another. Their father was American Indian, and each of them were born on the reservation in Shawano County, Wisconsin.

I never met that grandfather. He died at a young age. His throat was cut, and he bled to death in a drunken bar fight. My grandmother wasn't much better and dropped my aunt, uncle, and mother on the doorstep of different relatives' houses from Wisconsin to Tennessee. You see all things work together, and later my mother was sent to Sparta, Tennessee, where she and my father met. He was enlisted in the Air Force and was home to attend a funeral where my mother was also. They met and were soon married and began a new life 500 miles away.

Remember in chapter one, how you can pass down traits and even disabilities to your children? Well, my parents were workhorses, and that easily passed down to me. During these days of the Mississippi life, my grandparents, who owned the farm, had pretty much raised nine children, and they had all got off that farm as fast as they could. They married, moved, and joined the military. A single farm with nine kids meant free labor for at least twenty-five years. Now my grandparents were struggling with no help, and on a weekend call home, my father made the choice to uproot his young family and move back home to be poor and become a workhorse again. It must have been tough for them both, because they had already buried their first son (my oldest brother) in a section known as baby land under a tree in Biloxi Mississippi.

They moved back home, and in the next couple of years that followed, they would bury their second and third sons side-by-side under a different tree in Sparta. All my parents ever wanted was a large family, and here they were, living in poverty in middle Tennessee as workhorses for my grandfather with one child a lifetime away and the other two close by but impossible to embrace. A few years later, along came my sister, then me, and then my little brother. Did you catch that? Not only was I the middle child, but I was also the oldest son. I was custom-designed as the middle child, and in the years that followed, I was groomed to be the next workhorse. I did a more than adequate job carrying on the family tradition.

The workhorse was a natural fit for me, and I did it pretty well. There's something that I learned in those days that has stuck with me all my life, and that is, people will follow a leader that's in the ditch with them

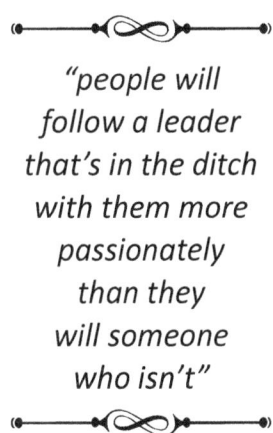

"people will follow a leader that's in the ditch with them more passionately than they will someone who isn't"

more passionately than they will someone who isn't. Craig Groeshel says people would rather follow a leader who is real than one who is always right. My parents never told me to work; they went with me and showed me. They stayed with us until the daylight was gone, and when one of us left the field, we all left together.

In the book of Genesis, two brothers find themselves at great odds. They were twins who looked nothing alike and were as different as daylight and dark: Jacob and Esau. The story is widely known and preached about Jacob stealing his older brother's birthright resulting in a young Jacob fleeing far way to escape his brother's wrath. Well, all things work together, and Jacob spends the next fourteen years as another man's workhorse. Jacob had the favor of God on his life and every time his father-in-law Laban would cheat him, the Lord would bless him even more.

Jacob was even lied to and deceived into marrying the wrong sister. He was in love with Rachel. She was all he really ever wanted, and he gave seven years of his life as a workhorse for Laban just to earn the right to marry her, only to find out the whole family created a sting, and the older Leah was slipped in as the bride. Jacob spent seven more years laboring for his father-in-law just so he could marry the woman he fell in love with to begin with. Sometimes all we want is an honest return from an honest day's work, not a rusted-out old water tank.

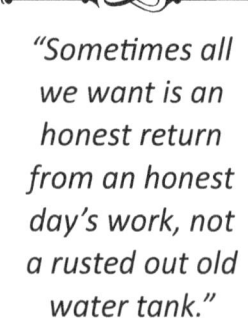

"Sometimes all we want is an honest return from an honest day's work, not a rusted out old water tank."

Several years before I was born, my great uncle on my mother's side had a house that he built on a hill away from others. He was fairly wealthy and hired my father to hand-dig a water line to his new house on the hill. It would have to be below the freeze line and several hundreds of feet long. He told my father that he would "make it worth it to him." My father took one pickaxe and a shovel and ran a water line hundreds of feet through crag rock, limestone, and hard clay by hand, and when he finished, my uncle gave him a rusted out water tank and fifty dollars as payment. He saw a workhorse and took advantage of it. To him, he may have thought fifty dollars was adequate payment for such a job, and it may have been. But my father felt under-appreciated. I'm sure the water tank was just a gift. It impacted my father to the point of mention several times in my life growing up.

The other horse in this chapter is the packhorse. He's a lot like the workhorse except this guy gets worked to death but never gets to carry the rider. His job is to carry the gear and supplies for the cowboy. He's tethered to the rider with a strap. He walks in the same footsteps as the rider's personal horse, but he does it with his head down. Here's the sad part: nobody ever notices the packhorse. He's the one you work to death because you know he can carry the load.

Surely you've watched a western or two. the cowboy sits upon his noble steed as the wind blows through the mane of the stallion. He raises up on his hind legs, and the world notices him in all his grandeur. Are you seeing the picture I just painted? You didn't even notice the packhorse cropped out of the scene, did you? And when the bad guys start to shout at the cowboy on his stallion one of two things happen; he drops the leash from the packhorse and rides into the wind with bullets blazing and guns drawn. And two, he jumps off of his personal horse, slaps it on the backside, sending it away. He grabs a rifle and uses the packhorse as a shield against the onslaught of gunfire. Are you following me, camera guy? The packhorse is dispensable.

Like I said, the workhorse comes natural to me, but I have felt like this packhorse many times. In the late fall of 2006, my pastor, who I loved, came to my house, sat on my couch, and asked me to become the associate pastor of the church. He wanted to let me know that in the distant future, he would be retiring, and he wanted me to learn and love the people and step into his role as pastor once that day came. Of course we were very honored and excited. We accepted, and a new season in our lives began. For the first time in my life, I had a pastor who loved me for me, not for the work I could get done or the pack I could carry. We worked even harder, and two years later we went on staff full time.

The days soon winded down three years after, and on the day of one of my granddaughter's birthdays, he pulled to the front of my house and informed me that he was officially retiring and his last Sunday would be only a couple of weeks away. Of course I thought it was time for me to step into the lead pastor role, but there was a catch, we were part of a denomination, and state leaders could care less what conversations were had on couches five years earlier. My wife and I had become the workhorses for twelve years. We loved every step of the journey but were passed over and never considered for the job. Did I feel like the job should have been mine? Yes. Did I feel under-appreciated? Yes.

> *"state leaders could care less what conversations were had on couches five years earlier."*

Did we later get our chance to lead pastor that church? No. It was over, and soon a new pastor arrived. His first words to me were, "I don't need you, I don't know where I can use you, don't ever speak on my behalf, and I guess I am going to have to cut your salary." Once again, a nine-second statement just placed a period at the end of twelve years of work. He was the stallion, and I was the packhorse. Packhorses can be replaced. After all, he was the new pastor. The job wasn't mine, and it never would be.

But here's the problem with the packhorse. He carries almost everything. He's mostly unnoticed, but when he's gone, everything seems to go with him. We knew that God was leading us out, and this time we knew he was calling us to lead pastor. The problem was, we didn't know where or when or even if that would ever happen. We began to interview and try out at churches across the state of Tennessee, but something was happening during those tryouts: they didn't want us, either.

We were a bit too progressive for the style of churches they were sending us to. So we continued working and packing and soon realized it was time to tap out. I was part of the worship team and had been for several years. Now I stood behind a new pastor who really didn't want or need me, and God subtly spoke to my spirit one afternoon and told me my time there was over. We moved the next week to the balcony and began to plan our departure. But the problem with the packhorse is that he carries all the stuff. Our fingerprints were on everything.

Lots of people were there because of our connection with them, and we soon realized we couldn't stay, but how would we leave? There's only one way to leave, and that's the same way David did when Saul threw spears at him. David left alone. Sure the packhorse carries a lot. And sure, there will be a giant hole when he's gone. And yes, maybe that person even has connections with people that could affect the church. But nevertheless you leave alone.

People may not stay, but you can't be the one they follow. We left and sat at another church just waiting on God to open a door. Any day now he's going to give us a church. It surely will only take a few weeks—a month at the most. Nothing happened. Every once in a while we would try out somewhere, and yes, they would reject us.

Here we were in our late forties, shepherds without a flock. All we needed was a flock without a shepherd, but where do you find one of those? After all, you're just a ditchdigger from Sparta, Tennessee. You're the son of a ditchdigger. You have no pedigree for ministry and actually you have no one who even knows who you are. All you need is for someone to put you in the game.

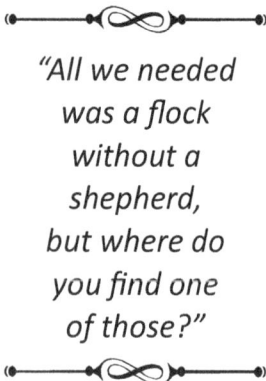

"All we needed was a flock without a shepherd, but where do you find one of those?"

There's one thing about workhorses, once they get in the game they'll play harder than anyone else. But ditchdiggers can't pastor churches.

Sometimes the journey is not as bad as it seems. But it's hard to be reminded of that while you're in the middle of it. Jacob spent fourteen years as a workhorse, but during that time, God was doing something in him that I'm not sure he even noticed. He was growing a family and also becoming wealthy in the process. God promised his grandfather Abraham that he would become the father of nations and that his offspring would be too numerous to count. He had two sons as an old man, and only one was the rightful heir. His son Isaac only had two sons, and now we find Jacob fathering the heads of the twelve tribes of Israel, all while he was living and existing as a packhorse.

What Jacob may not have realized is that as the packhorse, he was not only carrying the master's burden, but he was also cultivating his own anointing. Jacob's story also has a *but* in it. "*But*" I robbed my brother of his blessing. "*But*" I tricked my father. "*But*" my name literally means deceiver. Jacob has a lot of *buts* in his story and now he was about to have another. On the eve of his long-feared encounter with his brother Esau, Jacob did something in the dark of night that would unpack his horse and change his life forever.

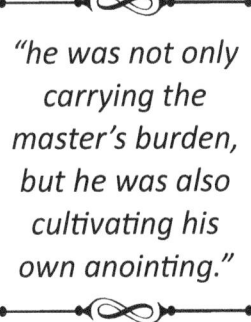

"he was not only carrying the master's burden, but he was also cultivating his own anointing."

He would spend the night wrestling with God until God had to dislocate his hip just to get him to let go. God unloaded the pack that night. He set the workhorse free and literally changed the way he walked for the rest of his life. Now he has a brand new *but* in his story.

"Oh you're just Jacob, the deceiver.

"Yes I am *but* that's not my name anymore; my name is Israel."

"You're just Laban's workhorse; you can't lead a nation."

"That's true, *but* I don't walk the way I used to, either."

We can always find a reason not to obey the Lord. Maybe it's time for you and me to spend some time with God and get a brand-new *but* in our stories.

We felt sent out by God to pastor a church, but like I said, where do you find one of those? God sent us out from where we were and—no one wanted us. Plenty of churches wanted the workhorse, but they weren't lining up for the stallion. So we waited and kept working where we were. Then one day after almost two years, I remembered a word that was spoken over us almost three years earlier. "God is not calling you to the north, south, east, or west; he is calling you from within." Why had God brought that to my mind after all this time? Maybe we weren't supposed to go to another city or town. Maybe we weren't even supposed to lead pastor. Maybe we were just simply supposed to be the workhorse for someone else. After all, we were at a new church and under a wonderful pastor. That's it! We were called to stay where we were. So I went straight to him the very next service and told him our new revelation and that he could count on me! His response was that he was starting a new Wednesday study and needed my help. Finally after almost three years of rejection, I was going to be accepted as more than a workhorse. I was going to be asked to lead a study. This has to be what God was waiting on.

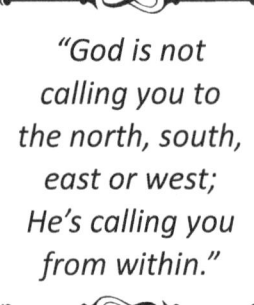

"God is not calling you to the north, south, east or west; He's calling you from within."

My heart was overwhelmed with excitement and then it came: he had the perfect spot for me. He needed someone to play the part of a mad scientist on a weekly basis. He wanted what everyone else over the past twenty years had wanted. He wanted the crazy and goofy Steve. He wanted me to be the hype man, not the teacher. To this day he doesn't know what that did to me. I don't blame him at all.

It was absolutely 100 percent God. God knew I was about to settle into another workhorse role, and he wasn't about to allow it. I was so excited for a brief moment and then went home and cried. For the first time I told my wife that if this is ministry, then I didn't want any part. I had reached that point. We were in love with the Lord but not so much with the people, and it didn't take long for that old familiar nine seconds of rejection to rear its ugly head.

The next Sunday, we sat in the very same service that I thought a few days earlier would be my landing spot, and I was the most miserable person in the house, surrounded by wonderful and loving people and I felt like I was at a party I wasn't invited to. I knew "there was more." The next day as we backed out of our driveway, I stopped and just simply told God, "Either fire me or put me to work." A few days later, a church in town without a pastor that had already called once, (and we turned them down) called again. This time God had our attention.

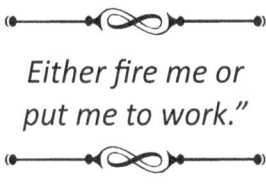

Either fire me or put me to work.

They were a flock without a shepherd. We were shepherds without a flock, and God had said three years earlier that He would use us from within. We met with the entire church around a single table on a Tuesday morning. It was unanimous; we would give it a whirl. Our first service would be Mother's Day 2013.

We showed up. That was a huge step given the circumstances over the past few years, and you know what? None of the people we had ever ministered with or to showed up. We reached out to three unchurched families, and they came. That first Sunday, we brought more people than they actually had attending, and as they say the rest is history. We will dig a little deeper in this story in the following chapters because as Paul Harvey would say, "There's more to the story."

Jacob must have spent many days thinking, *There's more.* I'm sure he thought of it when he would look at the relationship between his brother and his father. Did he think of more when his brother and father would laugh and reminisce over the day's hunt as he would watch from a distance? What went through his mind that first night after leaving home, when his head lay on a stone and his eyes gazed at the stars? I like to think his thoughts were, *There's more*. Every time his father in law would try to cheat him, and he faithfully clocked in for work, his mind surely thought, *There's more*.

Jacob became the father of each of the tribes of Israel. His son Joseph saved the whole family, and God multiplied them. All of this was made possible because Jacob knew his role as a workhorse in the early days. Even when he knew there was more, he still continued working and packing for someone else. He waited patiently, and during that wait, he served faithfully and honestly.

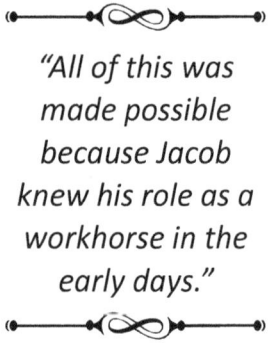

"All of this was made possible because Jacob knew his role as a workhorse in the early days."

So you're tired of serving your boss or maybe your pastor. You're exhausted as a workhorse. You've even asked, "When's my breakthrough coming?" In the meantime, don't despise the journey. Your desire may not be to serve coffee or greet folks at the door. Your heart may be to teach a class or join the worship team. *There's more* doesn't mean there's nothing to do until I get to do what I want to do. It simply means enjoy the workhorse role until that teaching job opens up. I was a workhorse for many years—actually all my life, and I enjoyed and cherished almost every minute.

There's more horses to visit. I'll see you in the following chapters.

Chapter 3

THE MUSTANG

Three seconds remains on the clock. Here's the inbound pass, and there's the drive to the basket. The guard passes off to the power forward. He's up for the shot; he has a good look at the basket. Here's the shot and—it's good! It's good! Our high school basketball team had just won the district playoff and was state bound. We were the underdogs in a game we were not supposed to win. It was 1979; we were the visiting team, and the crowd went wild. Now before you start thinking that I may have been some hotshot star basketball player with a sweet jumpshot, let me assure you that is not the case.

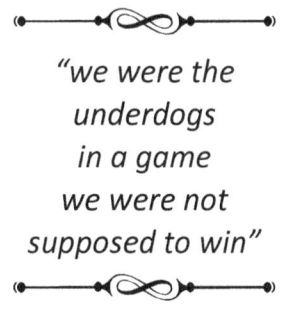

"we were the underdogs in a game we were not supposed to win"

I was there that night but not on the floor. I was in the stands as a sophomore. But before the night was over, I would play a greater role in the game than I thought possible. We had won the game as the visiting team, an hour away and on hostile hardwood. The gym was full of our folks. We convoyed a continuous stream of headlights from two towns away. We were White County, and basketball is the county religion. We're used to winning basketball programs, girls and guys alike. But every pack has a mustang in it from time to time.

That night the net was cut and held high in the enemy's backyard. Did I say the net was cut? Yes, I did, but not in the traditional sense. There was no awards ceremony. There was no customary eight-foot stepladder and a pair of scissors. No, there was a farm boy wearing worn jeans and a cap, with a razor sharp knife. The challenge was made, and I accepted. We were cutting the net down.

Did I mention that I wasn't a player? Did I mention that spectators aren't allowed to cut the nets? Yeah, we didn't know that. I was hoisted high and with one bold slice, the net no longer belonged to the home team. It was now the property of White County High School. But as quick as I was on foot, I was no match for the long arm of the law. As soon as my feet touched the floor, an officer's hand grabbed my shoulder, and off I was whisked. However I was not about to give up my most prized possession, so I tossed the net and open knife to a school mate, and off I went.

I was being carried out of the gym forcefully by an angry and upset local policemen. He had just witnessed his hometown team be eliminated from state contention. He had seen a long-haired, gangly kid cut his net down, and the jig was up. I was in some deep horse fertilizer. All I could think about was who I would call to get me out of jail. I surely didn't want to call my father or a relative.

The policemen must have had an affection for me because he held me tight as he crashed open the gym doors leading into a desolate hallway. He walked me down the hall of the school like we were newlyweds. Just as we were approaching the final set of gym doors, they suddenly flew open. And there to my wondering eyes did appear— my very own high school principal. Lord, shoot me now! I was only a sophomore, but he and I had spent time together in his office on many occasions. I would almost rather spend the night in the enemy's jail. He firmly stopped the officer and told him who he was and that he would deal with me severely. The exchange was made, he politely thanked the policeman, and we exited through the doors and back into the gym. At that point he patted me on the back, told me to have a good time, and sent me back into the celebration.

Some of my friend's fathers have mentioned "the net" incident for many years since. I'm told our school sports program was placed on probation because a wild mustang in a gym full of fans destroyed another school's property that night. The probation thing I'm not sure of, but one thing I do know is mustangs gotta run. Mustangs are the wild horses that just can't seem to find a comfortable place inside the fence. They're always peering over the edge of the corral and thinking, *There's more.*

The untamed character and personality of a mustang will always push him to run. He never finds himself seeking status quo. Coasting is never a long-term option, and few are ever able to tame him. He's simply a long shot. A poor bet. A loose cannon. Too high of a risk. You know the one; you can find him with very little effort. He's the one holding the tattered basketball net in

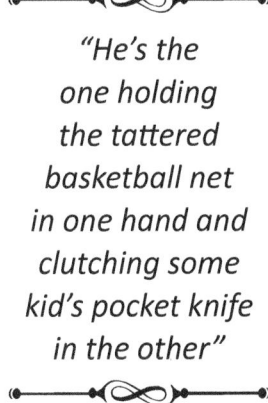

"He's the one holding the tattered basketball net in one hand and clutching some kid's pocket knife in the other"

one hand and clutching some kid's pocket knife in the other. That's the one.

You may find that you fit into this category fairly well. Be encouraged because Saul's son Jonathan was a mustang also. In the book of 1 Samuel, chapters 13 and 14, Israel is without weapons or even a blacksmith to make them. Saul is king, and he and his son Jonathan are the only two with swords. The Philistines are the enemy, and they have pretty much cut off all roads and passes. The mustang in Jonathan had gazed over the fence long enough.

The other team's court was right over there. All we have to do is go over, just me and my armor bearer. All we have to do is climb a steep cliff and win a battle where we're are outnumbered 20 to 1, Jonathan thought. Mustangs jump fences when no one else is willing to try. There is no way Jonathan and an unarmed companion can win that type of encounter from that much of a disadvantage. But you see, Jonathan knew someone the Philistines didn't. He knew his God as the source of great victory.

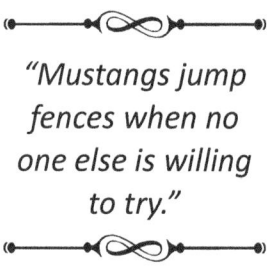

"Mustangs jump fences when no one else is willing to try."

Three seconds remained on the clock in an away game on hostile ground, and the Philistines tried a psychological bullying tactic; they talked smack to Jonathan and his armor bearer when they stepped onto the court: "Look, the Hebrews are coming out of their holes. Hey, the Hebrews are so scared, they're hiding." What the Philistines didn't know was, they were about to get their nets cut by a couple of mustangs. Jonathan and his friend climbed on hands and knees to where the Philistines were. Two men stood against twenty. Jonathan twisted, turned, and glided as he wielded his sword with laser accuracy. The enemy fell one-by-one behind him, the eyes of his armor bearer would be the last thing they would see on this earth. Jonathan and a single helper had done the impossible. God had used them to bring about a great victory for Israel.

Nets only get cut at the end of the game for ceremonial purposes, but this game was won when Jonathan began to gaze over the fence and say to his friend, "There's more." The enemy was defeated the moment they looked down upon a couple of mustangs with disrespect.

You might remember I mentioned that I was a ditchdigger, but I never told you how I went from the ditch to the pulpit. First of all, as far as I know I'm the only minister that my family has ever produced. I grew up in a conservative, overprotective home, but most of those years at home weren't Christian based. We were loved and well cared for, and that was more than most had. As I grew older, I just gravitated to the ditch. After all, that was my father's business, and one day I found myself in a ditch with my father's business partner, knee deep in water repairing a water main break. In the midst of the mud and heat of the day, my dad's partner took a chance on a filth-covered mustang and invited me to church.

Of course, I said yes. And of course I didn't go. And of course he didn't give up. It took several months, but eventually Tena and I went, and the rest is history, they say. Not so much. I left after that first visit and didn't go back. But eventually we did go back, and on that second encounter we gave our hearts to the Lord. At twenty-five years old, Tena and I both knelt at an altar on the left side of a little Nazarene sanctuary, and on the third Sunday in September 1988, we began a brand-new Christian walk. Somebody had taken a chance on a wild mustang, and I'm glad he did.

Victory at the hands of Jonathan and his armor bearer was the first quarter of a game Israel was supposed to lose, but that first quarter set the rhythm for the rest of the game. The Philistines had been smacked in the mouth, and they knew it. Momentum had shifted, and more victories were on their way. God had used the king's son to accomplish the impossible. A wild mustang who decided to run free had broken a hole in the stall for the rest to run through. Now, please don't misinterpret the heart of a mustang. Jonathan wasn't rebellious; he was daring and visionary. The mustang spirit is never a blank check for rebellion. True mustangs aren't rebellious; they just know how to run.

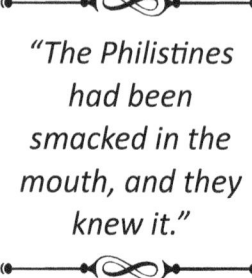

"The Philistines had been smacked in the mouth, and they knew it."

Our lives were forever changed one morning under a doorway at that little church when I felt "the call." I had never experienced anything like that before, but I knew what it was. In an instant, God had shown me the direction my life would take for the next seventeen years. I was going to be the next youth pastor of that church. There was just one problem. There was already a youth leader in place, and they wouldn't be giving up that spot for a wild mustang to take over. I immediately told a lady standing next to me, and she politely and firmly told me to forget it; it wasn't happening. But I knew the job was mine. You see when God calls you to a work and someone else is already there, it's only a matter of time because they can't keep warm at someone else's fire.

I only spoke about it to those closest to us, and everyone encouraged me to believe but discouraged me that it would actually ever come to fruition. I would circle the corral and gaze over the fence, and for the first time instead of thinking there was more, I knew there was more. There was one person that bought the vision, though, and it was my wife Tena. We were young, but we knew what we had to do. However, the lady who occupied the youth leader's seat was in my way. I loved and respected her, but she was warming her hands by my fire. The job was no longer hers; she was absorbing someone else's anointing, but I wasn't sure she knew it. It felt like she had held that position for a hundred years.

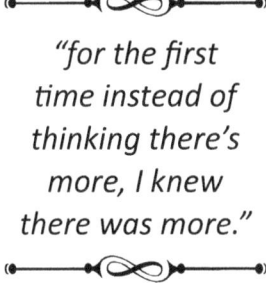

"for the first time instead of thinking there's more, I knew there was more."

One of the few I spoke with was the pastor. He was relatively new and continued to encourage me. Three months later, he called with news: this lady's husband had taken a position in another town and there would be an opening available very soon in the youth department if we wanted it. A few weeks later, Tena and I officially became the youth pastors. It would be an identity that we would own and cherish for almost two decades. We had gazed over the fence and knew there was more. Our first youth service, we stole a kid from the children's department and filled the room with a whopping six kids, two belonged to the pastor, two belonged to a church leader, one was the son of the church secretary and the other a friend of one of the other kids. We were six, but once again, we gazed over the fence and knew there was more—more teens, more lives that needed to be changed, and maybe more mustangs. A couple of months into the ministry, we took those six to a youth gathering of competitions in everything from sports to creative writing and Bible quizzing.

Once again, I knew there was more, and we knew we would return to that competition the next year with the largest group and a winning attitude. God called, and He equipped us. Our six soon grew into seventeen, and we moved to a larger room. Then we were thirty, and we rented a gym and for the next several years, thousands of kids came through the youth ministry. We had filled a gym with mustangs for years. Some of them were young horses no one else wanted. A friend had taken a chance in a ditch years earlier with me, and our gym was now filled with the same mud-covered mustangs who just wanted to run.

Sooner or later that kid that no one wants is going to ride in on the church bus. He may be a bit on the wild side, the one who marks on the walls and gets mud on the carpet. He's the one who disrupts class and is very familiar with time out or the rough kid who is quick to fight and slow to apologize. But he's the one who keeps coming because it's the one secure and constant spot in his life. He's the one who always takes another plate or steals a third and fourth cookie from the hospitality counter. He clogs the toilets and locks the stall door from the inside and climbs under just to be mischievous.

I sat in the hall during time out with that kid one night. I was called to speak with him about his behavior. We sat on the floor side-by-side, two mustangs, one young and one old (at least he thinks I'm old). "Nobody understands me," he said. We sat there in the hallway talking. I told him about a young mustang not so long ago that turned out to be the pastor of the church. He didn't need to be told how bad he was; he just needed to know how awesome he could be. You don't throw something away because it's has a few broken parts.

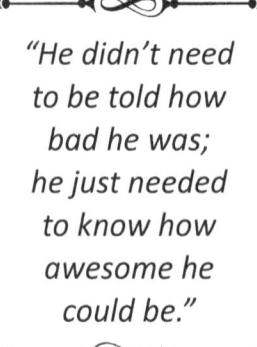

"He didn't need to be told how bad he was; he just needed to know how awesome he could be."

The Mustang

How many mustangs are sitting in our churches, in our homes, and maybe in the very chair you're sitting in right now? Let them run because that's what they were built to do. They're easily recognized if you try; just look through the crowd, and you'll see him. He's the long-haired, gangly one holding a tattered basketball net in one hand and some kid's pocket knife in the other.

Chapter 4

The Lead Horse

I grew up on a small farm, and there were times my father would take me back to the old-school way of doing things. He would hitch a mule or horse to a plow or some other implement. I would often ask why we would take the time to use an animal when we had a perfectly good tractor thirty feet away. He would always respond that "It's never safe to venture too far away from what got you here." During those times of "going old school" I learned terms like single tree and double tree. A single tree is a bar made from wood placed behind the animal that is attached to the horse and then to the implement or wagon for pulling. A double tree is the same thing but is designed for two horses.

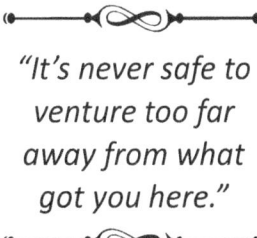

"It's never safe to venture too far away from what got you here."

I learned that young horses need to be taught. They need to learn the master's voice and be obedient to his commands. They are taught best by a good lead horse. The lead horse is located at the front left in a team and teaches the rest from that position. He knows the master's voice; he understands and obeys his commands. He passes down his knowledge from that position.

Every individual needs a lead horse in their life. Even the most powerful of warriors can find their roots running through a lead horse's harness. Allow me to introduce you to Joshua, the son of Nun. He was a mighty warrior and leader of Israel. He has an entire book in the Bible named after him. Joshua led Israel across the Jordan River and into their promise. Under his leadership, they conquered the impenetrable Jericho with hardly more than a shout; they defeated multiple armies and angry giants. They were a nation of worshippers. They were what I call the Joshua generation. But every leader needs a lead horse in their life. Someone has to be the one who passes down what they know, and without Moses, there would have been no Joshua.

The Lord built the platform that Joshua stood on, through his servant Moses. In the book of Exodus, chapter 19, the recently delivered Hebrew slaves found themselves at the foot of the mountain of Sinai. At this point they were just a large group of slaves. They were not yet a nation. They became a nation when God gave them the law from the mountaintop. A super-sized family had just spent the past weeks witnessing the hand of God strike the Egyptian king with unimaginable plagues. They had followed Moses through the Red Sea and watched as those same waters destroyed the enemy behind them while they focused on their God before them.

Moses is their lead horse, and the lead horse is always teaching. In verse 3, Moses begins to move up the mountain toward God. At that time, God called to him. This was a learning opportunity I'm not sure the people understood. It's also a perfect opportunity for each of us today. If we want to know what

The Lead Horse

God is saying, then we must start moving toward him. The closer we get to him, the clearer his voice becomes.

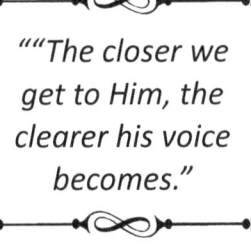

""The closer we get to Him, the clearer his voice becomes."

Who is your key man? You know, that "Moses" in your life from whom you can learn? Who's that one who can teach you, not so much by what they say, but by how they move, act, and react. You know, that one person that you just want to absorb from. Who's your lead horse?

I like to describe the Joshua generation as worshippers. The first thing Joshua did before crossing the Jordan was call the whole of Israel to consecration. They worshipped. You may find that you are more worshipper than teacher, your passion out-thinks your reasoning, and those moments of tarrying in the presence of God are what you live for. That's great, but never forget that Joshua knew how to worship. The times he spent in the shadows of the Moses and God meetings were created because of Moses. Joshua was there because of the doors Moses opened to the throne room to begin with.

My wife Tena and I have had the privilege of working with young leaders for almost thirty years. We have stood beside and ministered with some of the most anointed young Joshuas. However, for a brief time, we found ourselves in an unfamiliar place. Some of our young leaders began to find their own "tent of meeting"; they would spend time in a dark room with worship music playing just absorbing the presence of God. But out of those encounters, an attitude began to develop. Suddenly what was a unified church body became "us" and "them." They had discovered the market on worshipping God. They labeled the mature saints as the Moses generation, and the finger-pointing erupted.

I heard ideas expressed, like, "The older generation knows more about God, but we know how to worship Him." "The older folks are the Moses generation, and they need to learn how to worship God." *"They need to learn how to worship God!"* This broke our hearts. Our church had experienced steady and healthy growth under the leadership of our pastor for several years. He took the church when no one else wanted it. In the early days most of the people had left, and those who remained were in heavy debt with very few people to afford the bills let alone pay a shepherd. But those few people stayed the course, my pastor came on board, and they began to rebuild what had been severely damaged and left for dead.

Now a little over a decade later, the church was flourishing. Tena and I were the youth pastors with a large core of young leaders, some of whom thought they needed to teach these saints how to worship. The young colt suddenly doesn't need the lead horse any longer after a few hours of training. We quickly went into repair mode. It was our role and responsibility to fix what was broken. After prayer and planning, we realized what we had to do; we needed to get the Joshua generation harnessed closer to the lead horse than ever before. Therefore, we took these young worshippers and joined the main church worship team, and I went with them.

We plugged in our guitars and amps. We brought voices and drummers, and without knowing it, they were tethered to the lead horse. It only took a few weeks for them to begin to know the heart of the team. The Moses generation wasn't so bad after all. We became a team that respected one another because old

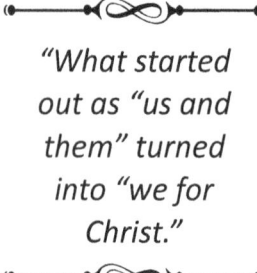

"What started out as "us and them" turned into "we for Christ."

and young alike worked together. What started out as "us and them" turned into "we for Christ."

The Word says that Moses went up Mount Sinai to receive the law from the hand of God Himself for the people. He was eighty years old. The word *Sinai* means "to shine, or divine truth"; some say the word means "sin." He went up. Moving up means the journey is still in progress. There is more to accomplish. But at the end of his life, when he was one hundred and twenty years old, God took him to Mount Horeb and he stood on the top and viewed the promise from there. The word *Horeb* means "the sword."

God bookended the last forty years of Moses's life with two mountain experiences. One was to bring the glory that would shine to cover Israel, and the other was the sword that would bring the battle for the promise. Your life and my life are a series of mountain experiences. We live our lives from pinnacle to pinnacle, with valley moments scattered in between. Moses was that lead horse for Joshua, and without his guidance, the promise would have likely remained just a promise. The conquest of the Promised Land didn't start when Joshua crosses the Jordan River. It began on Mount Sinai forty years earlier when Joshua was tethered to his lead horse. Great victories aren't always won on the battlefield; sometimes they're won on the practice field.

"Great victories aren't always won on the battlefield; sometimes they're won on the practice field."

In 1999, I was a proud member of the Joshua generation. I was a good and very passionate worshipper of the Lord. I had met Bob Robbins several years earlier when I was a young servant volunteer in my denominational church. I was given the opportunity to support our local church on a state level as a representative for that department. Every quarter, state planning meetings were scheduled in which I would attend to represent our church. That's when I met Bob.

As I have mentioned, I was always a misfit in such gatherings. After all ditchdiggers don't pastor churches, nor do they represent their churches in meetings. But the sessions were a breeze compared to the worse part of the day. *Lunch* was inevitable. There was no way around it. You have to eat, but no one ever said you have to invite the new kid to go with you. I didn't know anyone and they didn't know me.

I felt uncomfortable to invite myself into their circle or ask which restaurant they were going to, so I resolved to eat alone. However, Bob was the kind of guy who wasn't about to let that happen. Bob had been around for a while. He was a lead horse, and he tethered himself to a ditchdigger. Bob and I became friends, and I soon found myself looking forward to the quarterly meetings rather than dreading them. I genuinely liked Bob, and what was so encouraging was that Bob liked me. He was older than me, respected, and more experienced. Bob was a lead horse, and lead horses don't look back. They don't have to. They know the master's voice, and they simply lead.

"Moses didn't lead people out of something bad as much as he led them to Something great" "

Moses didn't lead people *out* of something bad as much as he led them *to* Someone great; he moved them toward God with every step. But notice with me that Moses didn't look back; lead horses don't have to. That's what I call a rearview mirror mentality. Are you that person who lives in the rearview mirror? Lead horses don't look back, and they especially don't live there. Fear lives in the rearview mirror. Moses led his people continuously toward God, not away from fear. Moses didn't even look back when he found himself trapped between a great sea and a furious Egyptian army.

Fear will always turn heads, and when I close my eyes, I can picture those millions of people looking back because that's what fear does. But there was one man who didn't look back, and that was the lead horse himself. They don't have to; they know the voice of the Master. Moses looked forward to the sea. He focused on a dry path that God established before He even created the water to cover it. God opened the waters, blew the ground dry, and Moses tethered himself to his people and led them where many would fear to go.

Moses's job was never to win battles. He didn't carry a sword; he carried a stick. His job was to teach a young nation to put God first. God before battle, God before conquest, God before triumph, and God before victory.

> "Moses's job was never to win battles. He didn't carry a sword; he carried a stick"

The year 1999 rolled around, and I hadn't seen Bob Robbins in a few years. God had led us out of the denominational church the year earlier, and so our paths just never crossed again. Tena and I had thrown ourselves into our business for that time, and part of that was baptistry repairs. So I got a call to repair a baptistry from none other than the maintenance guy at Bob's church. It was a two-hour drive for me, so we obviously weren't in the area very often. We discussed the issue on the phone and made an appointment to do the repairs the following Tuesday. Before hanging up, I grabbed the opportunity to ask about Bob, thinking I could maybe arrange lunch with him while at his church.

I was devastated to hear that Bob was fighting an aggressive cancer and wasn't expected to live very much longer. This was on a Wednesday, and that night while at the church I was attending, God began to speak to my heart with instruction: "Go to Bob's house and lay hands on him." I was overwhelmed with every kind of emotion. First of all, I didn't even know where he lived, nor did I know anyone in his family. I only knew my friend, but God said go lay hands on him. This is when it got real, "Go lay hands on Bob next Tuesday, but here's the catch, nothing but God until then."

Was I hearing God correctly? You want me to lay hands on a man that I haven't seen in two years, in front of his family whom I have never met, and to top that, in order to prepare myself for this task, I have to disappear for five days with no outside contact or interference? Yes, that was exactly it. Cancel and reschedule all my appointments for the next five days and replace it with silence and solitude—no work, no play, no family. That Wednesday night, I wept openly in that back corner of the sanctuary alone. God was calling me to do something I wasn't sure I could do.

Thursday morning came, and of course, I honored my work commitments. And there was morning and evening, the first day. On Friday morning, the sun rose, and I found myself being a good business owner. I showed up and made all my calls that were scheduled. And there was morning and evening the second day. Saturday was the only break I had, and my family deserved to have their father and husband spend quality time together. The weather was beautiful. The yard received a manicure, the shrubs were trimmed, and the beds weeded. And there was morning and evening the third day.

Sunday is the Lord's Day. We always serve him on the Sabbath. Church depends on us being there. And there was morning and evening the fourth day. Mondays are always so busy; it's traditionally the heaviest work day with the volume of calls alone. I'm not sure how much money I made that day, but I'm sure it was plenty. That part I don't remember because something else was on my mind. And there was morning and evening the fifth day.

"Tuesday's coming, are you ready"

"Tuesday's coming, are you ready?" Like it or not, it's coming tomorrow morning. It's all I had thought about for five days. How do I do something I'm not prepared to do? If I only had more time because Tuesday's coming. Tuesday did come, and in the eleventh hour, there was a reprieve. I had been saved by a flat tire.

Bob's town was across the time zone and was an hour ahead, and by the time I get this tire repaired and on the road, it would be too late to make it, so I did something to them that I couldn't do to the others the past five days and that was to call and reschedule. I was unable to reach anyone, so I left a message that I would have to make it another day, and I would follow up in a few days to reschedule. I think I felt a little like Jonah when he didn't want to do the one thing God was calling him to do. Jonah got a fish, and I got a flat tire, but somehow I felt as swallowed up as he did. Later in the week I was able to make contact with the maintenance man again, and we agreed on a new date to repair their baptistry. We talked a bit and I apologized for

"Jonah got a fish, and I got a flat tire, but somehow I felt as swallowed up as he did"

having to reschedule from our previous Tuesday appointment. He assured me it was quite alright and proceeded to inform me that Tuesday would have been a very bad day anyway because Bob died on Tuesday.

My heart sank. Bob had died on the very day I was supposed to lay hands on him. Tuesday came, and I couldn't give God five days of putting *God first* to know what it's like to spend a few moments in the shoes of men like Peter and John. Five days for God to show me that I was a good and passionate worshipper but a poor servant. I knew how to worship, but I didn't know how to put God first. Five days that could have changed the lives of Bob, his family and friends, and me. But there was something I realized through all of this, and that was that God only told me to lays hands on Bob and how to prepare myself for that encounter, but he never said he would heal him. God never told me he would heal him because he knew I would never go. I was a young Joshua, who was a good and passionate worshipper but was not yet ready to be the lead horse.

Well I made that second appointment promptly, and the very moment I knelt down to inspect the baptistry, I cut my knee badly on a piece of sharp metal. We stopped the bleeding, bandaged the wound, and I repaired the baptistry. I drove home, went to the doctor, and was sewed up. I got five stitches. There's a big scar on my knee to this day with five stitch marks, one for each day I failed my friend. It's a lasting reminder that obedience is better than sacrifice. It's a lasting reminder that God doesn't need five days, but I do. It's a lasting reminder that Tuesday's coming—are *you* ready?

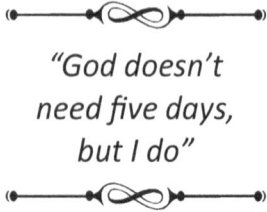
"God doesn't need five days, but I do"

There's one last thing I would like to mention concerning the Moses generation, and that is to remain tethered tightly to your lead horse. Honor that person, whether it be a mother or father in the Lord. I love my pastor with all my heart. Without him, there would be no Pastor Steve. Moses poured into, passed down, and catapulted forward into Joshua. Moses led two-plus million slaves from poverty and bondage to become the greatest nation on earth, but I don't think he ever longed to lead a movement as much as he longed to see God. But out of his passion to see God, he led a movement that is still growing to this day.

In 1999, I was without a lead horse in my life. I had recently lost my mentor, who was that person for me. I needed someone to tell me that I needed to put God first for five days, even if they had to pay for a hotel room themselves. I was a good and passionate worshipper then, and I still am today, but the only difference is that today I'm also confident in being the lead horse. Joshua became that lead horse after faithfully serving Moses for forty years of his life. There is no other path to the lead horse position. If someone were to come to me now with a five-day call from God, I would get them in a hotel room and their meals delivered to the door three times a day. I would instruct the hotel staff that that room is a "do not disturb" zone for the duration, and if they needed anything to call me. Maybe I will get that opportunity one day, and I hope I do because Tuesday is always coming my friends.

Chapter 5

THE MARE

There's the filly, and then there's the mare. The difference is the filly is defined as a female horse below the age of three, while the mare is over that age. I chose the mare for this chapter because of her wisdom and maturity, and I will be using my wife Tena as a role model for those same reasons. Now some of you may be saying to yourselves, "This guy sure is bold to use the terms *wife* and *mare* in the same vein of thought. Well, I didn't say old mare or heifer, so cut me some slack, and let's roll on."

Tena and I met on December 16, 1985. You may wonder how a person can remember the exact day when they met a total stranger. We remember that day very well, and as we continue, you will learn why. I was a few hours into my first day on a new job when there she was. However, the thing that caught my eye wasn't her stunning appearance. It wasn't her beautiful green eyes that I couldn't take my eyes off of as she spoke. I didn't even notice how beautifully and professionally she was dressed.

There's several more details I didn't notice during our first meeting at the sales counter that day, but the one thing that I saw as she walked toward the door was her confidence. She carried all five feet, two and a half inches like a commander of an army. That one moment still plays out in my mind today every time I hit "the replay" button. Picture it with me: she pulls into the parking lot, wayfarers on, and walks straight toward me, the wind blowing through her hair, I'm pretty sure I can hear Roy Orbison singing "Pretty Woman" in my head. Maybe I'm varying the details a bit, but little did I know I was standing toe to toe with my future wife. Someone has to be the strong one. Someone has to take the role of the mare.

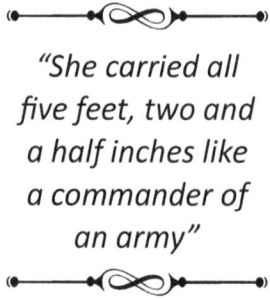

"She carried all five feet, two and a half inches like a commander of an army"

A couple of thousand years ago there was a family that lived in Bethany just outside of Jerusalem comprised of a man named Lazarus and his two sisters, Mary and Martha. One sister gets the distinction of being remembered and forever spoken of as the great worshipper and anointer of Jesus. Mary poured everything she possessed on her Lord. She even broke the jar, leaving nothing left to fill and exhibiting complete brokenness before the Lord. Now, if you notice, either Lazarus or Mary always gets the attention. But what about Martha? I think she gets a bad rap from many of us.

In Luke's gospel, Martha worked feverishly to serve. She prepared and organized the meal and probably cleaned the mess afterward. She did something that we should all learn from; she went to Jesus with her complaint rather than a bystander. She took her frustrations and disappointment to him. In chapter 10 and verse 40, she straight up asked Jesus,

"Lord, don't you care that my sister has left me to do the work by myself? Tell her to help me!" How many of us have opened a dialog of frustration with a coworker, ministry partner, or leader instead of going privately to Jesus? Yes Mary was the center of attention and Martha the complaining sister, but remember, most likely Martha was the more grounded one, the mature mare.

I think too many times we want to pick which sister we want to be, the passionate, carefree worshipper or the organized complaint-filled servant. Here's the catch: they both possessed the same DNA. Being the responsible one doesn't make you less of a worshipper or even a few degrees south of passionate. Likewise demonstrative worship doesn't make you "no good" for anything else. The mare possesses the DNA of the house, both the passion and security of Bethany. Without Martha, there most likely would not have been a meal, a meeting, or an open invitation, and without Mary, we wouldn't be telling this story today.

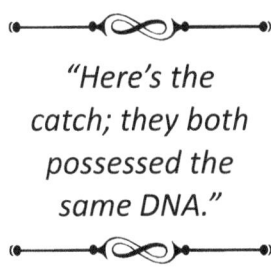

"Here's the catch; they both possessed the same DNA."

The woman I met at the counter that day possessed the spirit of Bethany. I saw a Martha confidence before I ever knew there was a Mary heart. I'm not talking about a false confidence that's found in beauty, although she has every right to that, too. I'm talking about a confidence in who she was as a person. As I write now at this moment, the Bethany DNA has been evident in my wife today, she started her day off at the feet of Jesus pouring everything out in prayer. Now she is meeting with a church volunteer to take care of an issue before it gets out of hand. Don't be so hard on yourself if you seem to see more Martha in your heart than Mary at times. Jesus needed both. Jesus loved both. Jesus depended on both, and we need both today.

Now I have a best friend that I talk to every day. As a matter of fact, I talk to my best friend all day long. My best friend is the one who ultimately introduced me to Jesus. Like I said, she stands a whopping five feet, two and a half inches tall. (That half inch is important and can't be left out.) On an overcast day in December 1985, we began to talk. It was my first day at the local electronics store.

Back in those days, the VHS industry had taken off like a rocket, and when I wasn't selling VCRs and stereos, I was supposed to help at the counter, renting videos. I wasn't sure how much freedom I had to spend with a single customer, but on this first evening on the job, around 4:30, I didn't really care. I was engaged in conversation with the spirit of Bethany—Mary and Martha all rolled into one. I knew I was going to see and talk with her again. After all I was close friends with her sister, so I knew I could get her home number from her if I needed to. Second, I had already been once bitten, and I just couldn't get that girl off my mind. You see she's just like her mother in every way.

It's the Bethany DNA. Tena can love with everything she has one minute and set a person straight the next. She can run corporations, manage households, pay bills, cook dinner, change diapers, and lead a Bible study and prayer time without batting an eye. Yes she is a chip off the ole block, just like her mother. But I never met her mother because the very hour she was returning her mother's rented video on my first day of work was about the time her mother was dying in a car accident. I had met the love of my life, but I would never meet the woman who made her what she was. I would never meet the prayer warrior that I only have grafted images of.

Over the next twenty-four hours, the spirits of Mary and Martha would have to take their position at the front of the line when the time called. Her mother was on life support in one hospital and her father on life support two hours away at another. She was the oldest child and the only person who could make a life-changing decision. On December 17, 1985, my not-yet-wife, made the choice at twenty years old to remove her mother from life support. The Mary in her wept and cried before the Lord for a miracle; the Martha in her did what had to be done. She made the decision to set her mother free to be where she had always longed to be.

Being the responsible mare doesn't mean you have to be perfect or even have a perfect past. There's a king who wants to make a difference in your life. He knows your past but doesn't disqualify you because of it, and neither should you. He doesn't see you as you are—He's a carpenter, and He sees you as you can be. You're saying, "But you don't understand; I'm a woman. Women don't lead." Yeah and ditchdiggers don't pastor churches, so let's look at John chapter 4.

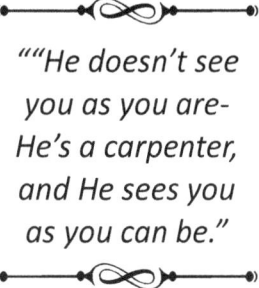
""He doesn't see you as you are- He's a carpenter, and He sees you as you can be."

Jesus deliberately met a woman who thought she couldn't lead, either. Jesus and his disciples were passing through Samaria when He did something outrageous. He stopped at a well with no way to extract water and sends his team on ahead of him to get lunch. He intentionally chose to stop at this time of day. He chose to be alone, and He intentionally chose this location, every plan, and every move, all because a woman would be coming at noon to draw water, and he knew it. Just a simple mare with a distorted past. We don't even know her name, but what we do know is that she doesn't like people.

She was gathering water in the heat of the day at an hour when she knew the well would be vacated. But on this day, there's one man present, and he's alone. Maybe one guy can't be too bad. Remember, she doesn't like people. It's not because of her personality but because of her guilt. She has a very questionable past in the community. She's sleeping with men to whom she's not married. That kind of lifestyle garners an image of rejections and shame that brings the atmosphere of guilt. It's just easier to avoid people.

That's why Jesus is alone. She wouldn't have proceeded that day to the well if she had noticed it full of disciples. "That's just more people to make me feel worse about myself than I already do." But Jesus has a different idea for, and opinion of, this lady. He wants to use her in a powerful way, and it's not just for a drink of water. He tells her who He is, and He reveals to her who she is. The culture of the day divided the Jew and Samaritan with hatred of one another. Jewish men didn't speak to Samaritans, and they especially didn't carry on conversations with Samaritan women alone. Not only was she a Samaritan and a woman, she was also a lady with a questionable past. She didn't have what you would call a favorable résumé.

She just wanted to get her water and get out of there, Jesus spoke first, simply asking for a drink of water. He went rogue by speaking to her, totally off Jewish script, and before the conversation was over, she was a changed individual. She left there and ran straight into town to spread the good news. Now this

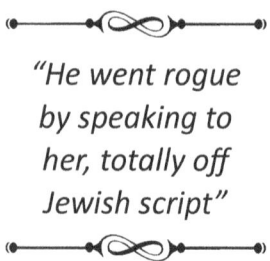

"He went rogue by speaking to her, totally off Jewish script"

was a woman that avoided people at noon, and now at 12:30, she's spreading the gospel to the very people she spent her live avoiding. You may be thinking, God can't use me *because I am a woman, or because I have a past.* Yeah, and he didn't use a shameful, embarrassed, and guilt-ridden lady to become one of the first evangelists of the New Testament, either.

You may say, "Even though I feel called by the Lord, women simply have no voice today." Think what you want, but it looks to me like Jesus doesn't call us and not equip us. And it looks to me that, as a woman, you already have a voice because Jesus made sure of that in John chapter 4, sitting alone at a well when he gave a voice to a single woman to save her town. Yes you have a voice. It was given two thousand years ago. It's not a voice of equality or a platform for political agenda. The voice God has given to women and men alike is to spread the gospel. It's the only voice that has the power to change.

My favorite part of this story is when the Samaritan woman "left her water jar" to spread the gospel of Christ. You see that water jar was her lifeline. It was her connection to her source of life. Water was so rare of a commodity in those days that wells were a sign of wealth and independence. It's the one thing you could not do without, and she left hers to serve him. That water jar represented everything she hated, despised, needed, and couldn't change about herself. It was the one thing in her life that she couldn't do without but, at the same time, couldn't stand to have to use. She left it behind.

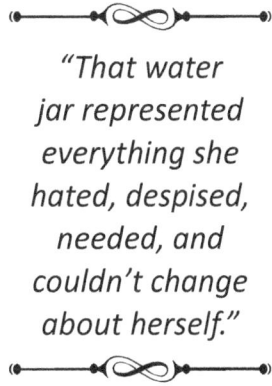

"That water jar represented everything she hated, despised, needed, and couldn't change about herself."

When we leave something behind, we are leaving a connection. She left knowing she would have to return. But her second trip to the well that day was much different than the first. The earlier trip was made with her eyes forward and head down. The second was to lead with vision. The earlier water jar represented her shame; the latter represented her freedom. People won't always go to the well because we ask, but they'll go when we lead them.

Time has a way of rolling on, and it didn't take long to realize that I wanted to marry the confident girl I had met in the store back in 1985. I did make that phone call a few days later, and we talked for hours. It was Christmas, and she was spending it without her mother for the first time in her life. Her father was still in serious condition and hospitalized, and maybe she felt a little like a Samaritan woman trying to fetch water. Maybe she didn't want to see anyone else. Maybe she was tired of being the strong one. Maybe she was all out of tears and just had no more to give. But she left something behind that connected us.

The mother-in-law that I never met had introduced me to the woman of my dreams. She had left something behind that connected us—a VHS tape. A simple plastic container with a roll of tape inside had been her water jar for her daughter. I don't know what she rented, I'm sure it was a sappy chick film, but it's the best movie of my life. That one video connected Tena and I. We were married six months later, but that's not the rest of the story.

My mother-in-law was a gospel singer. She had a beautiful voice, and she and my father-in-law traveled the southeast, singing and preaching through most of the seventies. She had a relationship with Jesus that few will ever possess and many long to encounter. Not only did that video connect Tena and me, but it also connected me to my Savior as well. Four years after we were married, my mother-in-law's voice began to reverberate in Tena's heart, and it was time to go to church. There was only one bump in that road, and it was me; I wasn't going. I didn't want Jesus or church, but that all changed one day, A few pews back in that little Nazarene church when Tena and I began to move toward Jesus.

You see ditchdiggers don't pastor churches, but try telling that to my mother-in-law. She believed in me even though she never met me. I cannot count the people I have prayed with to receive salvation. I fail to remember everyone we served with or the leaders we helped train and encourage. I'm not sure how many of them are pastors, evangelists, missionaries, and teachers, nor the marriages we fought for and broken hearts we cried with, but I know one thing for sure, and that is without that one video a thirty-nine-year-old mother left behind, none of that would have been possible.

The mare—she has no voice, you say? On the contrary, her voice is so loud it is still leading people today. It's not a voice of equality or political platform that lasts or makes a difference; it's the voice of salvation to the masses that never goes silent. So stop viewing your gender and your past by what you think it should look like. Stop disqualifying yourself out of what Jesus is wanting to qualify you into. Don't despise the water jar you've been given. Leave it at the well, and when you return, you'll see it completely different than when you left it. Videos and water jars speak louder than you think, you crazy mares.

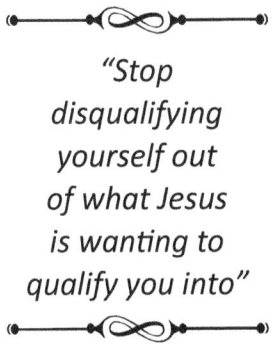

"Stop disqualifying yourself out of what Jesus is wanting to qualify you into"

Chapter 6

THE STRAY HORSE

According to a greendoor.com statistics, there are over 643,000 homeless people on any given night. No matter who you are or where you are in this world, everyone wants a home. In the late summer of 2011, Tena and I were blessed with a week away at a resort in Orlando, Florida. As we would reenter the gates each time, they would say, "Welcome home." Somewhere around the second or third day, the sound of welcome home permeated our spirits, and we knew God had just given us our new welcome statement for church. As an associate pastor, I was bubbling with excitement to tell my pastor what we felt God had laid on our hearts for our church. We were unofficially using a similar statement about home anyway.

The first chance I got after returning home from vacation was to speak with my pastor. I told him what was on our hearts, and he agreed with excitement and ordained a training session with our greeters. I was so excited to begin welcoming people home as they entered our doors. But there's always seems to be a catch; the next month my pastor announced his retirement. I tabled the idea for a month or so until the new pastor arrived. I was excited to talk with him about the new statement and genuinely expected the same enthusiasm I had received from my pastor several weeks earlier. That didn't happen the way I envisioned it. His words were, "Home is not a pretty place for some people, and they don't want to be there. We won't be using that statement as long as I'm here."

You see, God gives the vision to the head, and I wasn't the head. But why had he given "Welcome home" to me? What I didn't know then was that he had given it to me for Christpoint Church, not another man's church. I had a vision for a home I had never seen, a love for a people I had never met, and all I wanted was to go home, but it would be two more years before I would get there. We were stray horses. But why did it take two years? We knew God had called us home but we didn't have one to go to. Why wait two years? Why live like stray horses for so long? God has a reason why He does what he does and in the timing that He chooses.

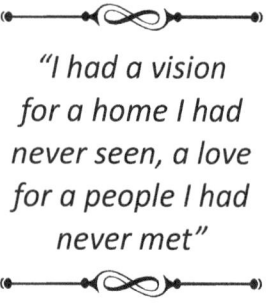

"I had a vision for a home I had never seen, a love for a people I had never met"

Why would God allow Israel to live in slavery for 430 years? Let's go back and see how they got there to understand one of the reasons He did what He did. The Old Testament is filled with strays. Abraham left what he knew to follow a God he had just met. He lived in a tent and believed in a promise that it seemed would never come. God has a way of using drifters and strays. Abraham held tightly to a promise of great multiplication during a time of barrenness. Sometimes God "stills" his people in order to expand them. He kept Noah in one place long enough to build a boat large enough to relaunch a civilization.

You may feel like a stray horse searching for a home that seems to never materialize. But one thing we can learn from God's stray horses is, home must be established in God before it can be established in location. Allow me to introduce you to Sierra who, at a young age, searched for a home in questionable places. The wrong boyfriend and the wrong attitude led her to follow a path that didn't lead home. One drink became two pills, and the process continued until she had spiraled into a hole she couldn't rescue herself from. She had established home in things other than God. Ten years of drug abuse and even prostitution had so altered her image of home that she had forgotten even the memory of what it was supposed to look like. I realized when I looked into her eyes what that pastor meant when he said home was not a pretty place for some people.

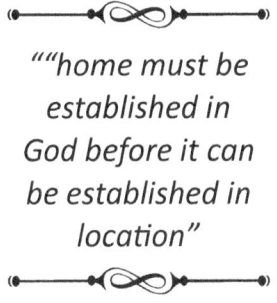

""home must be established in God before it can be established in location"

I realized that he himself had a distorted image of home. Maybe he had not yet established his home in God. Yes even preachers are not exempt from Satan's attacks. For Sierra, home would never be a place of peace and refuge without Jesus. She attends our church now with her husband and family. She's learning what home really looks like, and her image of home is beginning to fall into place. When we lack having a home, we lack security, and in that absence, we will try to substitute that loss of security with something that falsely fits. Drugs and sex abound, and the ones who are good at manipulation will cover their shame with haughtiness and arrogance. The difference is, the drug addict gets rejected while the arrogant gets excused. The sad fact is they're both longing for home.

Meet Kelly; her beauty is the first thing you notice when you meet her. She married her sweetheart when they were still kids. It was the first home she had ever known. Her parents had been married so many times to so many different people that her model for marriage had been severely skewed. Their young marriage had taken bumps and twist through ups and downs, and they added a few children as time passed. Kelly had a life, marriage, and children to share it with, but what she never allowed in was a home. She pushed her family in search of a home from state to state, job to job, and city to city until she finally asked for a divorce after twenty years.

Home must be established in God first because without him, the house will crumple. Kelly lived in many houses, but she never established a home. There was even a long period she spent serving the Lord. She became passionate for Him, but there is a difference between building houses and establishing a home. People live in houses every day, but they still feel homeless. Half of our marriages today are in failure not because of their houses; it's because they lack a home.

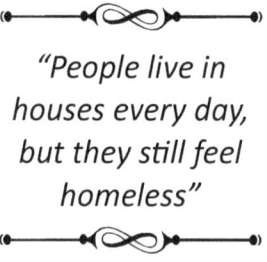

"People live in houses every day, but they still feel homeless"

My mother is a very strong woman, spiritually, mentally, and physically. She and I were the only ones in the room when my father's cancer diagnosis was elevated to a death sentence. One of us wept, and the other stood strong not to let her husband see her pain. She stood like an oak through fifteen months of treatments and the slow death of my father. She never let him see her cry, but I caught her weeping privately once. A few years later, we sat in a funeral parlor choosing a service for my sister. She had been suddenly taken from our lives by a drunk driver, and one of us wept again between the rosewood and baby blue casket options. My mother chose the rosewood with dignity.

Trials and tragedies came and went, and my mother stood firm. The only time I saw her shaken was a brief season when she unwisely co-signed for a loan that quickly became hers to pay. She became fearful that she could lose her home they had never owed on. Her security was threatened for the first time in my life. She worried and lost sleep over the idea of becoming homeless. The problem was solved in a few weeks, and life was quickly back to normal. My rock-solid mother had come close to becoming a stray, and it threatened her security.

Israel spent 430 years enslaved to Egypt. God originated their beginnings as one old man and woman past their prime. God gave Abraham his long-awaited and promised son. But one child named Isaac is a long way from a nation. Isaac only had two sons, but one of them was Jacob, and through him the heads of the twelves tribes of Israel were born. But twelve sons are still a far cry from "as numerous as the stars in the sky." God dried up the land and moved the nation of Israel to Egypt. He "stilled" them in Egypt in order to multiply them. A family went into Egypt, but a nation came out. Egypt was never their home. They would cross one body of water to get to freedom; they would cross another to possess their home.

Tena and I had a vision in our hearts and even a bold "welcome home" statement, but we had nowhere to call home. We knew what it felt like to be homeless, and we promised ourselves that we would fight for as many stray horses as we possibly could. At the beginning of our homeless journey, a lady spoke a word over us that God was establishing a place for us, but it wasn't going to come from the north, south, east, or west; rather, it would come from within. During our two years of homelessness we tried out and interviewed for churches in every part of Tennessee from the north, south, east, and west, but none wanted us. It took two years to meet the crew we would lock arms with as Christpoint Church. It was in our own town. It was within. We had almost forgotten about "welcome home," and the day we were to meet with "the six" to talk about launching a church, Tena informed me that she didn't want this and that she was against pastoring there. We walked in, and the first thing we saw was a sign that said "Welcome Home" (which is still hanging there to this day).

That was the moment she was no longer on the outside. She knew she was home. Our conversation with the prospective church members meandered through doctrine, personal testimony, vision, and expectation. Then one of the patriarchs said something that has reverberated within my spirit ever since. "If we fail to love people when they enter those front doors, then we have failed as a church." From that one statement, we knew we were home. Our job is to love them before we can lead them—to welcome them home where they can establish their home in Christ.

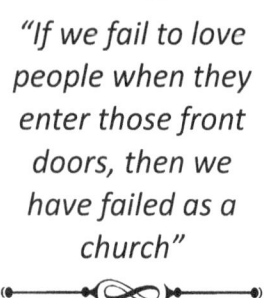

"If we fail to love people when they enter those front doors, then we have failed as a church"

The Lord has taught me not to despise the journey so much. We launched Christpoint church with six people and a vision, but our expectations were greater than our staff size. We wanted to grow exponentially, but God won't send us people to neglect, and we weren't ready to grow at that speed. We grew steadily while in the wait. People needed somewhere to call home.

The Stray Horse

David found his misfit warriors during the wait. I would argue that David's army was the greatest assembly of soldiers ever to enter the battle zone. In 1 Samuel, chapter 22, David escaped to a home in the ground. He'd been anointed king, but he had no kingdom. All he had was a cave. He was homeless. I guess you could call him a stray horse. But something happened in that cave: people were drawn to him. His brothers and his father's house joined him there.

Notice in verse 1 that it says his father's house and not his father's home. His father had a house outside of the cave but made a home on the inside. Then God sent David his army. The ones in debt, distressed, and bitter found themselves coming home. While waiting in a cave, David found his army, and they found their commander. Home must be established in God before it can be established in location. David spent a large portion of his early life anointed as king but running for his life. He had long since established his home in God; therefore, the location was only a formality.

During one of his escape routes from Saul, David ended up finding refuge behind enemy lines. You're truly the king of stray horses when you find that hanging out with the enemy is better than going home. In 1 Chronicles, chapter 12, David is behind enemy lines at Ziklag. Verse 1 shouts "stray horse" when it says "while he wasn't able to move." David was in a temporary dwelling because God had him at a point in life where he was unable to move. Please, my friends, let's learn from the great king David himself and know that even though we may be a stray horse at the moment and

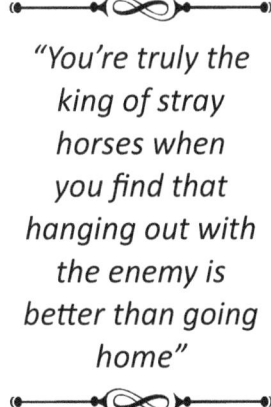

"You're truly the king of stray horses when you find that hanging out with the enemy is better than going home"

feel like we are homeless, God is still God even in the wait. God not only kept him from moving, He used that immobility to send him warriors and build his army. They were not just any soldiers, but "mighty warriors" leaders of hundreds and leaders of thousands.

Be encouraged, and know that although you may feel like a stray, you're not homeless nor are you alone. God may just be building your army while you're waiting. Maybe you feel like a stray horse because you've let someone's words take root in your soul and sprout seeds of abandonment and rejection. You may be reading this and realize that you feel like an outsider in your organization, workplace, or school. Maybe it's your marriage you feel trapped in. You think you're the only one trying and your house is feeling less like a home with every argument. Maybe you are the only single person in the group, and it doesn't seem that anyone will ever love you. Maybe you're fitting into any one or several of these categories. There's good news—David probably felt this way at his camp behind enemy lines also. Know this, if we are obedient to Jesus in the wait, then the warriors will come, the words will stop piercing, the marriage will heal, and your future is nearer than you think. You are not alone and you are loved.

Tena and I spent those two years in the wait much like David did. "Welcome home" was now a part of our DNA, but we had nowhere to apply it. We only knew one man out of those original six, and we had turned them down months earlier. Now God was leading us back. We didn't roll out of bed that morning, thinking of how awesome this meeting would be and how we would welcome everyone home. No, we went to that first interview, thinking it would be like all the others, that it would be just another opportunity to leave feeling alone and rejected, kind of like a stray. But the first thing we noticed was the sign hanging on the wall that simply read, "Welcome Home." After two years as strays, we had found our cave, we had found our warriors, and we had found our home. We are so conditioned to welcome home that it is part of our culture from the parking lot in. You can't say Christpoint without saying, "Welcome home!"

So you find that you may fit into the stray horse category, homeless in a room full of people, alone in a crowd, or just simply embarrassed by your past. You're in good company—father of nations, cave-dwelling kings, staff-carrying deliverers, and even a simple ditchdigging pastor. You have great value, and you're more wanted and needed than you think. Don't judge what Jesus can't do through you by what you see in yourself. Israel wasn't delivered in a day, and if God planned their exodus when they were still slaves, rest assured he's planning yours as well. Remember he's a carpenter, and carpenters turn raw materials into masterpieces and stray horses into thoroughbreds, so welcome home.

> *"Don't judge what Jesus can't do through you by what you see in yourself"*

Chapter 7

The Dead Horse

We've disclosed the fact that I'm the son of a farmer-slash-ditchdigger who was raised on a small farm in Tennessee. And those days on the farm produced mostly very fond memories. We were centrally located in the middle of our road (which is named after my grandmother), and we were surrounded by a few more equally small farms. Jimmy lived on the farm to the east that connected with ours. He was a year younger than me and was one of the few on our road, who wasn't a relative. We could either meet through the fields, through the woods, or just take the one-mile bicycle ride to one another's house. When our fathers didn't have us working, we would build forts, fish in the ponds, or wrangle the steers to the ground from the back of a horse. We were a bit reckless, but as long as we broke one of our bones instead of the steer's or horse's, we were okay.

We had reached the young teenage years, about the age of fourteen when we made a discovery behind his barn at the edge of the field. It was his father's mule, and he was dead. At first our minds wondered if we had inadvertently been involved in its demise and soon ruled out that option. We concluded that he must have just grown old and reached the end of a good life. Either way, he was DOA. Fourteen-year-old minds can do some pretty crazy thinking when unsupervised in an open field. It was simple math, one plus one plus one equals three. Number one, we have a dead horse. Number two, we have a perfectly good backhoe a mile away. Number three, "Let's bury this thing."

How convenient that this one day a backhoe was at home and not on the job somewhere. It must be a sign from God, so off we went. Now I could drive it but had really no idea how to operate it at this young age. I had watched my father many times as I helped on the job, so I thought, *How hard could it be*? I was fourteen, no driver's license, no prior experience, and no clue what I was doing. I had driven a ten-ton machine a mile on back roads, and now here I sit at the edge of my friend's field, gazing at two levers and a mule carcass. It was time to dig, and dig we did.

It took what seemed like hours to dig what I had watched my dad do in a few minutes, but we got the hole opened. It wasn't the prettiest hole, and as we soon found out, it wasn't the deepest either. We had done our good deed for the day. All we had to do was shove him in there and cover him up. But fourteen year olds have a high flaw capacity when it comes to depth ratio as compared to height restrictions; the hole wasn't deep enough. The poor mule's legs were too long, and they stuck out the top. He was already in the hole, so we couldn't get him back out, so we buried him anyway. We learned something that day, if you're going to bury your neighbor's mule, dig two holes, one for the horse and another for his legs. That was decades ago, and some wins that we took away that day were: My friend got his mule buried at no cost, and I got a crash course in backhoe operations 101 and a new perspective on depth perception.

The Dead Horse

When something is dead, that means that life is no longer present in that thing. Sometimes it's easy to recognize a dead horse (or mule), but other times they may not be so easy to spot. A guy once stood in a valley as a dead man; the only problem was he didn't know it yet. As a matter of fact, no one knew it except for one young, perhaps fourteen-year-old boy. A huge giant of a man known as Goliath was a fierce and tested warrior for the Philistines who were passionate enemies of Israel. They gathered their forces and drew their battle lines against Israel. The battle zone looked much like a ravine with steep inclines on each side, leading up to mountain tops that formed the valley below.

Israel assembled on one plateau and the Philistines on the other. The army that advanced first was at the greatest disadvantage due to having to pursue the other from the low point. So they remained in a standoff for almost six weeks. During this time, Goliath would challenge and insult Israel twice each day. He was a dead horse with a shout; he just didn't know it yet. All of the Philistines saw him as their champion, undefeated and unbeatable. The whole of Israel viewed him in fear and saw him as too powerful, too large, and too skilled to fight. They also saw him as unbeatable. Even the Israelite king, Saul, viewed the monolith in the valley as unbeatable. But one young boy saw him as he was—a dead man with a big mouth.

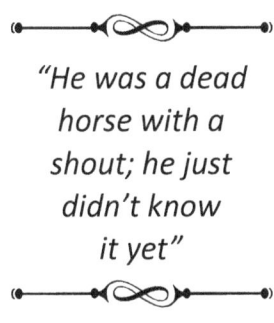

"He was a dead horse with a shout; he just didn't know it yet"

David entered the valley floor with nothing more than a few stones. Even face-to-face, Goliath didn't know he was a dead man. David even spoke to him to inform him of his fate, and he still couldn't see it. Goliath was a dead horse the moment he stepped to the front lines; he just hadn't finished falling yet.

David ran to him, struck him with pinpoint accuracy, and like I said, he was a dead horse. David removed the giant's head with his own sword. A kid from the hills had defeated the greatest warrior of their time with a rock. It's not always the biggest guy who wins the fight. It's the one who envisions the victory from the hillside, the only one who sees a dead horse when everyone else sees fear. That's the one who wins the fight.

In order for fear to take over, faith has to die. That's what fear wants to accomplish. It wants to kill our faith in God. David didn't kill that dude because he was better or because he was fearless. He killed him because he was faithful to know God. I'm betting when he entered the valley that day, he felt an element of fear. I'm also confident that he had already viewed Goliath, sized him up in his head, calculated his strategy, grabbed a handful of faith, pushed past the insults, and saw the Philistine's threat as nothing more than a dead man with a shout.

God has never called you to be the one struck with fear because of someone's shouts. He didn't build us with a "fear element." It has been said that babies are born with only two fears: the fear at falling and the fear of loud noises. Every other fear is one we have learned, allowed in, or permitted someone or something to place there. Paul empowers us in his second epistle to Timothy that God has not given us a spirit of fear. An old evangelist and teacher friend Mickey Bonner once told me that fear is devil faith. The very words we allow in that are not Godly and righteous for building will set up fertile soil for fear to grow. "You're not good enough, you're not smart enough, you're not." We let the "You're nots" infect and have control over the "God cans."

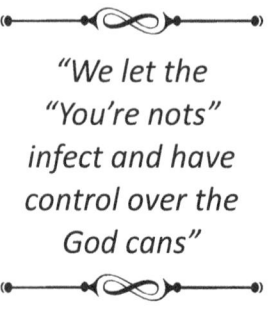

"We let the "You're nots" infect and have control over the God cans"

The Dead Horse

One of our most diligent servants at church has a crippling disorder that affects the long nerves in her legs and arms. I'm sure she has received multiple "You're nots and you can'ts" from doctors, friends, and family. Those words are dead horses to her. Her giant shouts at her every morning of her life, but she chooses to see them as dead words with no substance. Every morning, those words shout loud but are really dead; they just haven't fallen yet. But as her eyes open from her pillow and from the minute her feet touch the floor, she charges the hollow shouts and watches as her giant falls. The only thing I've found that she's afraid of are mice. Other than a rodent, everything else is a dead horse waiting to be buried.

Her husband has a "you can't" story also. He was told as a high schooler that he wouldn't make it in college and that he should choose a more technical or labor path. He graduated college, worked hard his whole life, and retired as a hospital administrator. He had to run toward his "you can'ts" every morning of his life to watch them fall. God beat terminal cancer in him when his giants screamed, "Give up; you can't win." He charged those voices every day through surgeries, treatments, and recovery. We're playing golf this Thursday. They said he wouldn't be able to do that, either.

A few years back, Tena and I were at a local restaurant and saw some old friends. We began to talk, and as always, the subject of church came up. My friend told me that when their pastor retired, they wanted to visit our church. I asked them how old he was, and at the time he was 87. She proceeded to tell me that he held so tightly to control that he actually led from a place of fear. He was so afraid of anything new changing some things for the better that he micro-managed until the many became the few, and the few became one family that remained. I remember this church as more vibrant a few decades ago.

His calling hadn't died, nor had his ability to preach. His passion for the lost was every bit as strong as it was then; he had simply stayed too long. He had a black-and white-vision in an HD world. Times had changed, and he couldn't keep up. He had overstayed his anointing. His effectiveness had died; it just took several years to fall. In the meantime, the church slowly disappeared.

In late 2012 Tena and I were asked to help a church in the neighboring town. The pastor was much younger than me and felt God had released him. He would be moving on. He showed wisdom beyond his years to know that if he stayed, he would be out of God's will for himself and the church. He knew he was absorbing someone else's anointing. He called me and wanted to slip us in as staff and allow the small congregation to get used to us; then he would move out, and I would move in. We never heard a yes or no from God, so we proceeded to test the waters.

We were asked what we felt needed work. They had maintained the same look, style, and number of attending members as they did in the seventies when my wife attended there as a little girl. Our response back to that question was "everything." We began to work together to tweak a few things starting with the worship style and culture. We implemented worship practices, and although it was a struggle, it wasn't terrible (well, yes, it was terrible), but then we broke the cardinal sin and called a planning meeting with a few leaders to foster and encourage excitement. That was a nightmare to say the least. With every attempt to step forward, we took two steps back into the seventies.

One lady spoke harshly and said, "The way we have been doing things has worked just fine for forty years. We used to have great services here." Then she contradicted herself with the next statement out of her mouth: "We don't know why people aren't coming anymore." I tried to help them see that if they would just change a few things to help people want to be there, then it would be a start. It was an epic failed meeting from the start; they had been there forty-plus years and never had an organizational meeting, and they didn't feel the need to start now. The last thing I left them with was a bold and loving statement because I loved them very much: "If you don't change, then you'll eventually have to close the church." Their church was already dead, it just hadn't fallen yet.

A year later the church was closed, and the property sold. You can't reach back and move forward at the same time. You may be saying, "How can God allow a church to die?" Well He doesn't. Jesus only spoke death one time, and that was to curse the fig tree in Mark chapter 11. He expects His church to be fruitful. Fruit is the only thing He judges. When

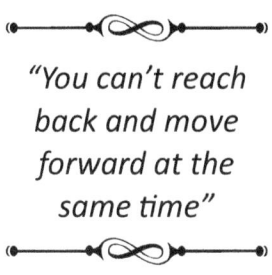

"You can't reach back and move forward at the same time"

he doesn't see that, then He moves on. He has no interest in pretty leaves. He's very direct in John chapter 15 concerning branches that fail to produce fruit. He also makes a bold stand in Revelation chapter 3 when He asked for the door to be opened when he knocks. Remember that in this passage, He's speaking to the church.

Saul became the first king of Israel and David the second. Saul was twice the physical man that David was but half the leader. About the only thing they had in common was the throne of Israel. God created man, but it's our job to establish our home in him. Saul was a fearful and self-serving leader. He was anointed king in the book of 1 Samuel, chapter 10. God instructed Samuel to take a flask of oil and pour it on his head. The next major event we see him is at his ceremonial crowning, where he was driven to hide because of his fear. On the contrary, David was anointed (as the last and youngest of his brothers) as king by the same prophet in 1 Samuel, chapter 16, but there's a difference. In verse 13, Samuel anointed David from a horn of oil, and the next major event we find him at is in the valley floor facing a giant that no one wanted to fight. Saul was anointed with a flask and then hid in fear. David was anointed with a horn and then defeated a giant. Something had to die in order for David to become king. The moment that ram was born, he was dead, but just hadn't fallen yet. That horn would be the vessel for David's anointing. Rams and lions, bears and giants, were dead; they just hadn't fallen yet.

Saul is the poster child for the dead horse. He could have been great fruit for the Lord and for the nation of Israel, but that wasn't to be. He became disobedient to the Lord's commands, and God rejected him. In 1 Samuel, chapter 15, God gave him the instruction to completely kill all of the Amalekites, including women, children, and livestock. He destroyed the weak and poor and kept the best as trophies, including the king. He was dead the moment he chose fear over faith; he just hadn't fallen yet. he served the rest of his life as God's rejected, a leader with no anointing.

When you're the dyslexic kid who can't read well, you know what it sounds like to hear the "you can'ts." They become very familiar words, and if the vision in you doesn't drive out the words on you, then dead horses are not far behind. Words are going to come, but how do we turn those dead words into living breaths of life? How do we call these things

"If the vision in you doesn't drive out the words on you, then dead horses are not far behind"

that are not as though they were? How do we turn dead horses into stallions?

God raised dead horses in the book of Ezekiel. In chapter 37, the valley floor was riddled with an army of bones. In verse 11, our bones are dried up, and our hope is lost. These bones are descriptive of dead horses. Hope of life is nonexistent. So how do we restore life to the dead horses in each of us? We have to speak life into them. Can these bones live? Then he said to me, "You have the power to speak life."

Chapter 37 gives us the recipe for restoring life to our dead passion, our dead marriages, our dead self-worth, and the dead places in each of us that have been made lifeless. While it's our position to speak life, we must remember that we are not the originator of life, and we are simply the conduit through which life is spoken. Jesus has already established that He is the way, the truth, and the life, so when we speak Jesus into the driest of bones and the deadest of horses, the rattling begins. Not only are we empowered to speak Jesus, when we do, we raise an army. And Ezekiel described that army as exceedingly great.

Ignore the hollow shouts that bring death, and know the very words the enemy wants to put on you are dead horses that haven't finished falling. They just need the way, the truth, and the life spoken into them, and that's our job.

Chapter 8.

THE DARK HORSE

The gate was slowly locked behind horse and rider. The field was set, and he was a seventeen to one underdog, a dark horse. The gates flew open on a sunny Saturday in May. The Kentucky Derby was underway. He soon found himself riding dangerously close to the rail. He was dead last in the field of sixteen. He knew he had to make his move but not too quickly. His horse was the classic example of ADHD. In past races, he became bored and lost focus while in the lead.

Running in fifth place, a long journey to the outside would be too risky and time consuming. He needed an opening, and there it was. He aimed his horse between two others ahead of him on the inside. He surged to the lead, and this time he would not lose focus. His name was Ferdinand, and he had just taken the lead at the coveted Kentucky Derby. He was the classic dark horse, his rider and trainer were both too old and considered past their prime, and Ferdinand had a reputation of blowing leads. But not this day. This day belonged to the underdogs. This day belonged to the dark horse at seventeen to one.

In the book of Judges, a dark horse emerges as a leader for the people. The Midianites had come against Israel and oppressed them greatly. They would attack the fields of grain, plundering and destroying them and leaving the Israelites without food for the immediate future as well as the coming months ahead. They stole from them their livestock as well. Israel became so afraid of the Midianites that they retreated to the mountains into dens and caves. They needed a leader to unite them as one, and as God has a way of doing, he chose the simple and small to confound the wise and the strong. God came to Gideon at a wine press as he was beating out wheat in order to hide from the enemy oppressor.

A wine press in those days is reported to have been a hole in the ground hewn out of stone or lined with plaster. Grapes were thrown into the pit, pressed, and trampled upon until the pit would be full of juice instead of grapes. Threshing wheat in the pit indicates Gideon was hiding from the enemy in a hole in the ground in order to harvest some grain for his family to survive. Notice that God didn't call those doing nothing and hiding out in the caves. He called someone who was already working despite the threat of possible loss.

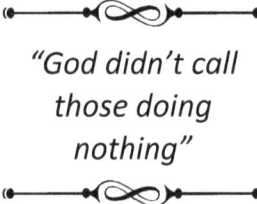

"God didn't call those doing nothing"

Now Israel had every right to be afraid of the Midianites. They were described as fierce, swift, and large in numbers—so many that their camels and tents blanketed the landscape and couldn't be counted. You're outnumbered, outpowered, outled and out-weaponed. And on top of that you're weak, starving, and mentally defeated. You're a dark horse, and even God had turned his back on you for a time. No one is willing to place a bet on you being able to stand against such an army. No one would even take a risk to incite such a rebellion. But God has a way of using dark horses to win races.

You may find similarity in yourself and the workhorse or maybe the mustang, but do you see yourself as the dark horse? I can relate so well with the racehorse Ferdinand. He seemed to suffer from a severe case of ADD. He just kind of lost focus as the race went along. He lost races because of his lack of focus. When we lose focus it's like losing "concentrate." Yes you read it correctly, I called it concentrate instead of concentration, and there's a good reason.

Back in 2015, I was working with one of my granddaughters on hitting a plastic ball with a plastic bat. At the time, she was only five years old. I would pitch the ball, and she would swing and mostly miss. After a few afternoons of practice, she got a bit more focused and became more successful at hitting, until— You see, she wanted to impress her Tete, my wife, with her batting skills and with the added pressure of someone watching, the desire to impress and trying too hard, she just couldn't make it happen. It eventually became too dark to see, and she was staying the night with us on that particular night. The next morning she woke early, came and got me, and wanted to practice before school. She said she had "lost concentrate" and needed to work on her swing to regain it.

Maybe you're like a five-year-old with a plastic bat- and you've lost concentrate. Because losing concentrate is the same as getting out of rhythm- and I did that in the last quarter of 2018. Our church had taken a severe blow. We had placed the wrong people in key leadership roles, who didn't possess the DNA and culture of the house. For the first time at Christpoint Church, we found ourselves out of rhythm. The problem with losing rhythm is by the time you realize it, damage can already be done. We struggled with losing people, and our giving plummeted for weeks.

Not only have you found yourself at a loss of rhythm, you've lost concentrate because of it, and when you look out, it seems like the valley floor is covered with tents and camels too numerous to count. The first few weeks we chalked up to a fluke thing. Just a few down weeks in giving. Twelve weeks passed, and we had went tens of thousands of dollars backward each month. First, I did two things: I tried to find out what was wrong and fix it, and I stood at my back door and cried. Here we were at Christmas time, and the entire fourth quarter had knocked our rhythm for a loop. Only a few staff members were aware of the severity of the problem.

We called a few people to meet and pray the day after Christmas. We have two campuses thirty minutes apart, and after intense prayer our hearts were broken. The new second campus prayer felt like victory. It felt like home. The main campus was the problem. We never felt a breakthrough. I stood in a corner, asking the Lord to give us what we needed that night, and I got my whipping as I prayed. He softly and firmly spoke to my spirit to stop asking for enough. "Start believing for more than enough. I am more than the God of enough so start treating me as such."

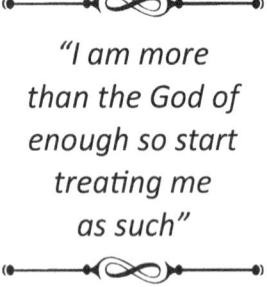

"I am more than the God of enough so start treating me as such"

We processed that for the next several hours, and finally what should have been the first option was actually the third. My wife said we have to call a prayer and fast, and we did. We believed for more than enough, and during that time God woke me up on a few occasions and flooded my spirit with instruction. On the morning of December 27, he showed me that we had lost rhythm and how to regain it. Our tuning fork had been touched and needed to be struck again. Our first service of 2019 had a different feel. There was a spirit of breakthrough we encountered even as we parked the car.

The familiar feeling that permeated the atmosphere of Christpoint Church since its beginning had been nonexistent for three months. Now it was back, and you could feel it, smell it, and taste it. That day during services, we turned off the cameras and live feed. We turned off the recordings and simply had church. We came together as a church body, locked arms, and prayed. Rhythm was reset in those services that morning. We had breakthroughs, and people got saved even into the following week. The Midianites had camped at our doorstep, and it seemed like we were outnumbered on every front—until that day.

God opened the floodgates, and what took us three months to lose, God gave back in two weeks. We heard from the Lord again and committed ourselves to fast and pray monthly. In the first week of April 2019, a husband and wife called the church, wanting to "donate some stuff." They gave to the church a building, extra parking lot, a new cargo trailer and diesel truck to pull it with. The combined value exceeded one hundred thousand dollars. A hundred grand from the Lord! Once again he showed us that He is the God of "more than enough," and He can do more with one percent of His planning than we can accomplish with a hundred percent of our own.

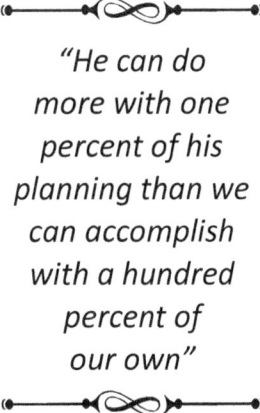

"He can do more with one percent of his planning than we can accomplish with a hundred percent of our own"

Gideon began his pursuit of the Midians with an army of thirty-two thousand men. That's a pretty large disadvantage to begin with. The enemy army was one hundred and thirty five thousand strong. That's a four to one underdog, but God had greater plans. Those odds were not good enough, so he reduced Gideon's army by twenty-two thousand, leaving the disadvantage at thirteen to one. Surely God knows what he's doing because he must be able to see something I can't. We're outnumbered thirteen to one, and we don't even have any weapons. Yes, God does know what He's doing. Ten thousand men was not a wide-enough margin, so God reduced His army yet again. This time, they numbered a measly three hundred.

God had not only reduced Gideon's men to one percent of what they began with, the reality was that the Israelite army which actually looked more like a large family were now outnumbered by the Midianites 450 to one, and God had the odds right where He wanted them. Gideon and his little band of warriors were the classic dark horse. How do you lead that battle charge? How do you rally men to know that all each one of you have to do is kill 450 skilled and more powerful warriors in order to win this battle? You give them a torch, a trumpet, a clay jar, and a shout. That outta do it. Gideon's army hid their torches with the clay jars and when the order was given they broke them, letting their light shine brighter than the sun. Their voices shouted for victory from a distance. Torches, trumpet blast, and shouts of victory pierced the darkness, and God made the sound of three hundred men elevate to the magnitude of thousands. The enemy turned on themselves in chaos and confusion, destroying one another. God had just accomplished the impossible through the improbable.

On that spring day back in 1986, I was busy working at the newly established electronics store. There were a few stores in the strip mall, including a grocery chain. In the five months of my employment, I had become friends with several of the workers from the strip mall. One came into the store and laid a sheet of paper in front of me to pay $5 and enter a random pool on Saturday's upcoming Kentucky Derby race. We would all pay five bucks and draw a horse out of the hat. You guessed it, I drew a seventeen to one dark horse named Ferdinand. Needless to say, I was the first to be surprised when my horse won. I had never watch a Kentucky Derby and wouldn't have watched this one if it hadn't been for the whopping eighty-dollar take home winnings I received.

What in your life seems to be that one thing that is too great to overcome? The one with the greatest odds against you or your success?

In 2011, I sat in the office of the state overseer of the denomination I was a part of at the time. We discussed the possibility of our being assigned a church to pastor or at least an opportunity to try out. I poured out my heart and visions for a church. He was cordial and polite and in my opinion secretly uncaring. I gave him the name of a church that I felt passionate about that was available, and that notion seemed to fall by the wayside. I distinctly remember trying to bring our dark horse image to the forefront. I told him that I realized he really didn't know us, but if he would give us a chance to pastor a church, we wouldn't let him down.

I think he took that to be begging, and so we left his office and were forgotten before we exited the building. We were outsiders trying to fit into a system we weren't made for. We were dark horses, hungry to get in the race, but maybe we were just trying to run the wrong race. We felt a little like Ferdinand; we just wanted to run. But there's more to Ferdinand's story than winning a few races. As he aged, he was studded out for several years until he was sold to a Japanese breeder. In 2002, the great Kentucky Derby winner Ferdinand was cast aside and sent to the slaughterhouse.

The heart of a winner resides in the spirit of the dark horse. The odds are always against him, but it doesn't keep him from running. You can spot him; he's on the inside lane, looking for that opening, that opportunity to surge ahead. He's unaffected by the odds against him; he just wants to run. He may lose a few races, but he keeps running despite the odds. The next time you view your situation and find yourself standing at the back door crying, remember God can do more with one percent of his planning than we can accomplish with a hundred percent of our own. Dark horses will never win derbies, and ditchdiggers can't pastor churches, but don't tell that to them; they like the odds the way they are.

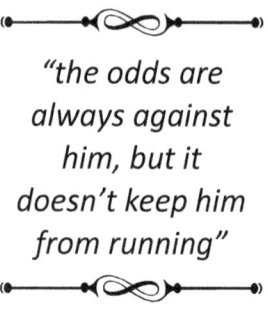

"the odds are always against him, but it doesn't keep him from running"

Chapter 9

THE TROJAN HORSE

September 29, 2018, is a day that will live in infamy, at least for Tena and me. That's the day she almost blew the engine in our car. Let's back up a bit, all the way back to January of 2017. In conversational dinner, something just kind of came out: another campus in another town. God had started a ball rolling in our hearts that in the coming days, He would be opening doors for a second Christpoint campus. But wait, churches in small rural communities don't launch multiple campuses; yeah, and ditch-diggers don't pastor churches either. Well, a few months went by, and the topic would resurface in our hearts or in conversation.

The next town over was the location God kept on our hearts, and we had no idea why. Neither of us was from there or knew anyone there, nor did we go there for any reason. But almost a year and a half later, there were several families attending our church from that community. So in May of 2018, we formed a launch team with plans to launch a second portable campus in the fall. We had a strong vision, but we had the wrong leader and the wrong team. What started out as a launch team quickly became a full-out purchase of an existing church and congregation. It seemed like a great opportunity.

We called prayer over our decisions and this merger. But what sometimes can look like the perfect plan may just be the perfect storm. We attempted to lock arms with the existing congregation, and in late June, we launched our first service at our new second campus. From that day on, we had a Trojan horse. What was working on the inside was more destructive than what we could build and repair on the outside. Tena and I were the lead pastors and visionary for Christpoint church (all campuses), but the inside was crumpling and being eaten away. We would walk into a campus that we pastored, and those old familiar feelings would resurface. We felt ignored, disrespected, and unwanted. We had an infection, and it needed medication real fast.

There's an insect known as the codling moth. It lays its eggs on the surface of fruit, undetected by the human eye. When those eggs hatch, the larvae will borrow through a small hole into the heart of the fruit. From there, it will destroy it from within. All the while the fruit has a healthy outward appearance. The fruit fly possesses a similar ability. It, however, pierces the flesh of the fruit, laying its eggs on the inside to start with. Ultimately, both outcomes produce the same results. They create a Trojan horse—defeat from within.

This is the same way the enemy wants to work in our lives to defeat us. He sneaks in through an unorthodox opening and sets up residence in the mind. He lays there patiently until his opportunity arises for attack. At that point, he's made his way to the inside, and he likes it there. After all, more damage can be done from the inside out.

Let's dig into the heart of two Bible leaders, who experienced a similar attack. Samson is the first leader to dissect. He was one of the judges of Israel during a time of great oppression at the hands of the Philistines. Samson was blessed with supernatural strength. He was bound to a very strict Nazarite vow that included not cutting his hair. Now we learn this story as children even outside the teachings of church, but let's take a look anyway. Samson had everything going for him. He was the Old Testament version of the man of steel. He couldn't be pierced or subdued. He had a vow with God, and no one could penetrate that shield. However, there was kryptonite, and it didn't look like crystal or possess a green glow.

Samson had a woman problem, not just a regular woman problem but a kryptonite woman issue. He loved Philistine women. He killed lions, ripped gates from their hinges, and killed thousands of Philistines all with his bare hands. Yet, he couldn't beat a small frail little woman. Philistine spears and armor were no match against the supernatural skin that he wore. However, he was no match for the oldest trick in the book either, a woman.

Delilah laid eggs of deceit on the inside. She bore straight into the heart of the Israelite warrior and destroyed him from within. How can something so small do so much damage? The codling moth larvae feeds on the seeds of the fruit. Even if the fruit ripens and falls to the ground, it cannot reproduce because the seeds have been destroyed. The enemy will enter through the slightest of windows. He wants not only to destroy our thoughts, but his ultimate goal is to destroy our future. The seed represents the future.

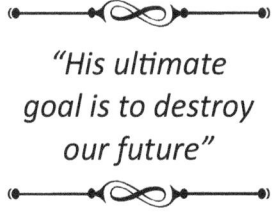

"His ultimate goal is to destroy our future"

The other case study for this chapter is Nehemiah. This guy had a bit of a different twist on a similar topic. You can read about Nehemiah in the book that bears his name. He was a cupbearer to the king of Susa when he received word of the great demise and shame of Israel. It was reported to him that Jerusalem's walls were in ruin and its gates burned with fire. This one bit of information set a fire in his heart to attempt the impossible. Was God calling him to head this rebuilding project? Was God anointing him leader over a people he really didn't even know? Has God called him to be more than a cupbearer? Why not him? After all, he had a position with the king. He had influence, and most of all he had the vision.

Nehemiah was granted permission to take that journey and lead the rebuilding of Jerusalem's walls. Without protection, they were vulnerable to attack. They were in a position of disgrace, and their future was unprotected. Nehemiah arrived in Jerusalem, and the first thing he did was to survey the damage. He actually had to dismount from his horse and walk over, around, and through the stones that used to be the walls of Jerusalem. Remember this lesson from the story of Nehemiah: everything that you think is destroyed in your life can be rebuilt. And not only is it rebuildable; all the materials we need to build with are not as far away as we think.

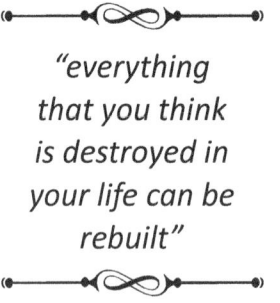

"everything that you think is destroyed in your life can be rebuilt"

Nehemiah had to crawl over the very stones that would be placed back in the wall in a few days. The enemy wants to kill, steal, and destroy, but in his haste to do so, he leaves the building blocks right where they are. He doesn't think we have enough faith in Jesus to start the rebuilding process. He underestimated Nehemiah, and he will underestimate you.

Nehemiah rallied the troops, and the wall was rebuilt in fifty-two days. But it didn't come without resistance. They were threatened on every front. Two guys by the names of Tobiah and Sanballat were the ring leaders and strongest voices against the rebuild. They attacked from the outside, unlike the Trojan-horse approach. The louder they cried, the harder the Israelites worked. The greater the threats, the more they banded together.

These two guys tried every tactic they could think of to attack the minds of the wall builders. This is great teaching straight out of the enemy's handbook. He starts with the voices that say you can't do it and shouldn't do it. Then he advances to a full frontal, "You won't do it." He works feverishly to convince us that our task will be a waste of time and that our work won't last.

There's a story our children and grandchildren are familiar with that provides a very clear parallel into our lives. There was once a husband and wife that lived happily with their many children in peace. One day when the father was away, an intruder broke into their home and killed all the children and the husband's wife. One child was spared, kidnapped, and carried off to a distant location thousands of miles from home. The father, distraught and overwhelmed with grief, set out to find the secret location where his lone child was being held hostage. The father had previously convinced himself and his son that to chase their dreams was impossible. He was alone, with no idea how to start searching or even what direction they went.

Early in his journey, he met his companion for the pursuit, who suffered from schizophrenia along with memory loss and delusional thoughts. Together they traveled thousands of miles to rescue the sole-surviving child only to find that he had perished at the hands of his captors. The father's name was Marlin, and his helper's name was Dory. In the end, the child who we know as Nemo was actually alive and reunited with his father, and they lived happily ever after. Nemo's father tried to convince him earlier that neither he nor his son could accomplish their dreams. He was convinced in his mind that they were too small and insignificant to do great things. Nemo refused to allow that

Trojan horse to set up residence in his heart. The dream was bigger than the fear of failure.

Now Tobiah and Sanballat couldn't shake Nehemiah from the outside, so they pulled a "codling moth" tactic and went to the inside. It all plays out in chapter 13, and we get the reasoning behind Tobiah and Sanballat's rebellion and hatred in the process; they were tight with the high priest. As a matter of fact, they were related to him and had distorted God's laws and statutes for a long time. They knew the presence of a new sheriff in town would disrupt and tear down their playhouses. Nehemiah left for a time, and while he was gone, the codling moth laid its eggs. Eliashib the high priest was the first to become rotten seed. He set up for Tobiah a residence in the house of God.

The priesthood and the temple were disgraced. Israel had reestablished their walls to restore their grace, only to find themselves disgraced from within. The ministry had been neglected during Nehemiah's absence, and worship had left the temple. The Sabbath laws were more than broken; they were a train wreck, and their Jewish bloodline and historical significance were being slowly diluted by intermarrying with the wrong people.

Notice with me that all of this happened while Nehemiah was not there. Nehemiah represents the presence of God for us today. Where the presence of God is absent, destruction will set in. Our lives, thoughts, and vision must be saturated in the presence of God for our dreams to come true. Move away from Jesus, and I promise something else will take his place. I would also like to point out that in the absence of Nehemiah, the Levites and singers had left the temple. Their

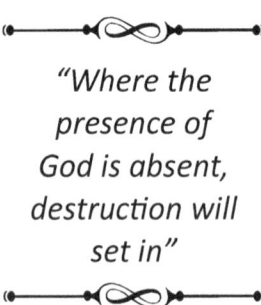

"Where the presence of God is absent, destruction will set in"

provision was cut off, and they were forced to the fields or starve. Worship had left the temple.

Today we are the new temples of the Lord, and where there's an absence of the presence of God, worship will starve. The opposite was true in the beginning when the wall was being built. They were under the leadership of Nehemiah, and the enemy was being starved out. As quickly as he mounted his horse to leave, the tides changed. Jerusalem had been invaded by a Trojan horse. But something happened when Big Poppa got back home; Nehemiah kicked Tobiah's sorry hide out, along with all of his furniture and belongings. He appointed proper leaders, brought back the worshippers and ministers, and redefined the sanctity of marriage. The Trojan horse attempt had failed at the hands of God.

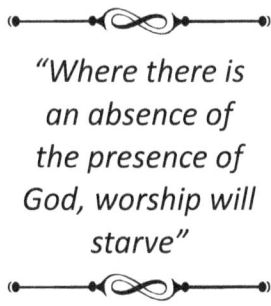

"Where there is an absence of the presence of God, worship will starve"

Now as we revisit the day Tena almost blew the engine in the car, allow me to catch you up. Christpoint Church was infected with a Trojan horse. This person had set his own agenda and esteemed himself as "the pastor" of a Christpoint campus. We had an Absalom spirit working on the inside, and it all came to a head in September. God had placed Christpoint Church in that town out of vision. This person felt he had spent long enough under our vision, and when he left, he took the new campus congregation with him.

September 29 was on a Saturday, and we had a satellite campus with no people left to attend. Yes you heard that right. Everyone was gone. Gene Edwards authored a book entitled *A Tale of Three Kings*, and in it, he gives instruction on the proper way to leave, and that is the exact same way that King David left when Saul threw spears. Later, he did the same thing when his son Absalom stole his kingdom through manipulation and deceit. Both times, David left alone. Leave any other way, and you are leaving wrong.

We called prayer for that campus, and on that Saturday, we attacked the Tobiah spirit and kicked him out. We anointed and prayed over every square inch—entrances, parking, grass, building, chairs, pulpit, you name it. We left, and I was attacked with one of those spears from behind as I pulled out. Within thirty minutes, I was on the floor writhing in pain. Now I have an extremely high tolerance for pain, but this was beyond that threshold by a mile. I was under attack, and I knew it. My wife rushed me to the ER for the first time in my life and, in doing so, almost blew the engine in the process.

I was rushed in, admitted, and quickly found that I was being attacked by a little intruder called a kidney stone. There was no reprieve, even in the ER. They gave one set of meds, and that didn't work. I struggled for several more hours until I finally agreed to try a second, more-powerful drug. I consented, and five minutes later I was in euphoria. I completely left reality, and in a moment of time I was in an apostle Peter-like trance. In that trance, I saw an extremely large black snake in a field of brown grass. He had the appearance that he was at least twenty feet long. His tail was toward me, and his head led straight to the chair of one of our prayer team members. It was the exact chair I saw her sitting in a few days earlier when I met with them. The snake was dark, and the ground around was dead and lifeless.

I quickly woke and went to the bathroom and passed the kidney stone. I was released and on the way home, stone number two made its appearance, and down I went again. Round two, and I had been knocked to the ground by a speck the size of a grain of sand. The Trojan horse was working on the inside of my body just as he had worked on the inside of our church. I was down for the count for the next twenty-four hours. I missed services that next Sunday morning, and our teams stepped in with grace and excitement to serve. We had scheduled a prayer celebration service at our main campus for that Sunday night at 6 p.m.

Somewhere around five o'clock, the kidney stone passed, and I showed up for service. I walked in, and the "head of the snake" was planning the service. For the first time since we launched, I felt uncomfortable in my own church. I felt like an outsider. I had empowered our prayer team to organize and conduct the service, and that night, we had a Trojan horse on the prayer team. That night she stood at the entrance to our sanctuary, instructing key leaders to leave our church. She said she was leaving, and so was the prayer team. She had been plotting with the former campus pastor behind our backs.

This spirit had to be dealt with immediately. We experienced a Nehemiah/Tobiah incident. The enemy had entered my mind that night. I felt like an outsider and even felt like I was being pushed out of the pastorate we had loved so passionately. Then one of our servant leaders went to the altar for prayer. I immediately knew why she was there and what she was paying for, and I went to her. I approached her as a defeated, sleep-deprived pastor with the feeling of losing his church. The second I touched her to pray, I heard that familiar voice from the Lord. "You're not a ditchdigger anymore; now rise up, and pastor my church."

Tobiah had been kicked out of our second campus, and now he was being kicked out of our main campus and out of my mind. God put that spirit out, furniture and

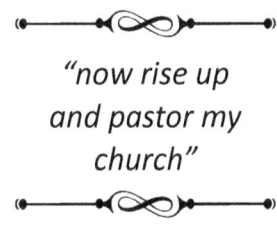

"now rise up and pastor my church"

all. But we still had to deal with the snake in the grass, so we did that the following week. On Wednesday, they met in the sanctuary of our church to persuade the others to leave. We confronted it head on. We fought to restore her and challenged her to ask for forgiveness and submit to Tena and me as pastors. She refused and took people with her when she left. We had lost everyone at the second campus, and now it had filtered home. Some of our leaders went to work and stopped the dam from breaking, but it would take another three months to find our breakthrough. That freedom came and was discussed in chapter 8.

Now I would be remiss if we left this story unfinished. We had service at the second campus on October 1, without anyone to fill the pews. We had been a week removed from that finger stuck in our faces and told we would not have church there. The infection had been removed, and now the body would have to be healed. We had met with leadership, and in a God-like way, we had just officially purchased and signed for the property. We were confident and passionate that God had called us there. he had committed us with a deed of ownership and a passion for souls we had never met.

That first service on October 1, one guy showed up. He was the director of a local halfway house where several men were transitioning to their next level of life. He gave his heart to the Lord that morning, and who did this guy start bringing with him to church? You guessed it, halfway-house residents, people that no one wanted, men and women with a past, individuals that society had labeled as rejected. The enemy had tried to defeat us from the inside out. No one was there to even show up for church on that first Sunday in October, but God sent the worshippers back home, and some of those people from the halfway house are now the heart of Christpoint Church. They are some of our most passionate servant leaders. That Christpoint campus is healthy now and continues to grow.

The codling moth larvae destroys the seed of the fruit. Seed represents the future. If we allow the enemy on the inside, then the seed will die. Give the seed to God, and He will multiply it, thirty, sixty, and a hundred fold. It's a no brainer!

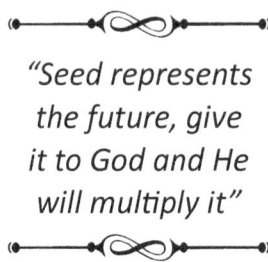

"Seed represents the future, give it to God and He will multiply it"

Chapter 10

The Pace Horse

God laid this book on my heart to write a couple of years ago, and I believe you are not reading it by happenstance. I believe he kept me from putting pen to paper because he knew the importance in the timing. The title, *More Than a Pace Horse*, was what resonated in my spirit. Yes, I grew up on a farm, and yes, I'm a country boy from Tennessee, but I actually have no history with horses. I really don't like riding them very much, either. I'm not very excited to sit on something that large that has a mind of its own. My idea of a horse being under me involves fewer legs and more in the way of two tires on pavement with my wife and me in the wind on some back road.

    I prefer to have control over my horses by twisting the throttle when I want to accelerate. I guess you could say I prefer an iron horse. With that being said, I don't want to offend the avid equestrians that may be reading this chapter right now, so I will say, I do love the elegance and beauty they possess. I value the great history between rider and horse, and I'm in awe when

I gaze upon them. I just want to leave the riding to someone else. But what about the pace horse? What's his story all about?

After researching the topic, I found the term I was actually looking for was *lead pony*. What I considered to be the pace horse was actually called a lead pony. The lead pony in horse racing terms is a thoroughbred that either didn't make it, couldn't live up to the hype, or has grown too old to compete. He is used to help train the racehorse to win. Every day, his job is to run side-by-side with the leader to push him harder and harder. In doing so, he teaches the money horse to recognize competition and to win. After all, a little competition always makes us run harder.

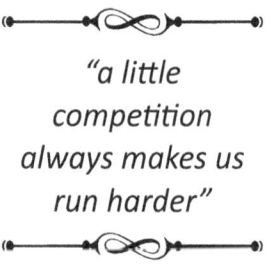

"a little competition always makes us run harder"

The sad irony of this matchup is that the lead pony was bred to run just like the money horse. He was gifted with speed just like the money horse. It's in his DNA to win, but he spends his days coming in second. He's trained to let the leader finish first. His life is designed around losing. He has spent the best days of his life shining a light on another horse. So as we continue, please know that when I use the term *pace horse*, I'm actually referring to the lead pony. The term of pace horse just seems to flow better as we read.

Take a look at yourself for a quick moment and see if the pace horse is you. But here's some points that are very important to remember: some people are perfectly designed to fill the role of a pace horse, and some aren't. Also, some journeys to becoming the horse out front must go through the pace horse. In other words, for some, you have to be comfortable being the pace horse for a season because it's the only way you're going to learn how to take the lead when the time comes. And finally, never underestimate the power of hard training. Running makes you a better runner.

It's kind of hard to pen an accurate model for the pace horse without looking at David and his best friend Jonathan. They were miles apart in their upbringing, but they were the best of friends. Jonathan was raised as the prince. He was a young thoroughbred who was bred to run and to win. His father was the king of Israel. He was a proven warrior on the field and a champion of many battles. Jonathon was raised to be the thoroughbred, and when you're the son of a king, you understand the value of running in second place. You know that as you serve, there will one day come an opportunity to step into the lead position. Jonathan had the pedigree. He was born to be the leader, and everyone around him knew it, but this guy was not your average spoiled rotten son of royalty. He was Jonathan, the one who knew how to run.

David, on the other hand, was not as we say in the south the ringneck pup. He was not the pick of the litter. David was not even the first choice of his father, nor was he the favorite. Why I would be willing to say that David wouldn't have chosen himself, either, given the chance? He wasn't even training to be a pace horse or a stable pony or anything else. He had no pedigree. He was the eighth son of his father and just a teenager at that. Then one day the prophet of God came calling.

Jonathan's father, the king, had disobeyed God's commands, and the Lord had rejected him. Samuel was God's chosen instrument to speak to his people, including the king. Samuel was tasked with seeking out and anointing the new king. God led him to the home of a man named Jesse, and it was clear that before he left that house, someone was about to be promoted

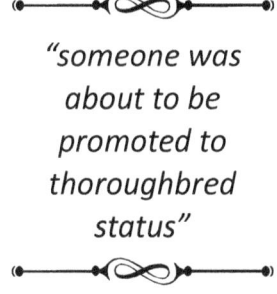

"someone was about to be promoted to thoroughbred status"

to thoroughbred status. Jesse invited all of his sons to the party except for one, a kid named David. One-by-one, strong young men from the house of Jesse were brought before the man of God to see which one would be the next racehorse. But each one was turned down until the room was empty. Surely God has not led Samuel here by mistake.

Surely he has misunderstood the Lord. Maybe we should run these guys through once more. They look good. They're healthy and strong and just simply look like thoroughbred runners, but—no they're not the one we're looking for. Then Samuel asked the question: "Is this all of your sons? Are there anymore horses in the pen?" "Well, there's this one more, way out in the field. We didn't bother to invite him to this meeting because we didn't think he was thoroughbred material."

Jonathan never got his chance to step into the lead role. He was second place to his father and then was skipped over to become a new second place to the rightfully anointed David. What makes Jonathan stand out is the fact that he was comfortable and totally content to remain a pace horse. He realized the favor that David had on his life. He had spent time with him, and David's personality and charisma had infected Jonathan greatly. Jonathan would forever remain in second place.

In the book of 1 Samuel, chapter 18, David has just killed the giant named Goliath. Jonathan and David's hearts were knitted together that day. Jonathan gladly accepted his role as the pace horse. He recognized the anointing of the Lord on David, and he stripped himself of his robe and weaponry and gave them to David, showing his commitment to serve the rightful king.

Some of us are built to be a pace horse, and Jonathan is the royal example of what he is supposed to look like. You may be in a subordinate role right now. You may feel like you deserve your shot at the title. You may even feel cheated and passed over because your time has not yet come. Look at Jonathan, and let's learn together that not everyone will rise to become the thoroughbred leader. There's only one way to step into this role, and that is to own it. Jonathan "stripped himself" of his robe. Our job as the pace horse is to strip ourselves of the self-proclaimed right to first place.

Strip ourselves of the pride and selfishness. Strip ourselves of the voices. Strip ourselves of our own vision, and submit to the vision of the thoroughbred. But stripping ourselves of these things still leaves us partially there. Jonathan then gave his royal robe to David. When we give away in this fashion, we are esteeming our leader by giving the one single thing that represents our royal position and that is "the vision." Here is my robe, David. It represents the future of God's kingdom.

The vision of the future lies with the wearer of this robe. When we serve our leader, there's only one vision, and that is his. Jonathan also gave David his sword, shield, and weaponry. He gave his tools for building. We have to be comfortable as the pace horse knowing there's only one set of blueprints, and that is the one God has given the leader for building. One more thing and that is, Jonathan gave David his means for victory. Jonathan won battles and was victorious by the sword. He willingly turned it over to David. In the pace horse role, your victory is submitted to the leader, and his victories become your victories.

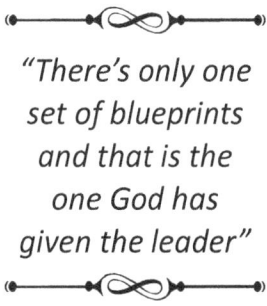

"There's only one set of blueprints and that is the one God has given the leader"

I personally have had many preachers in my life, but I really can only call two of those men pastor. I served under one as I was learning to walk with God in the beginning, but he wasn't able to stay around very long. The other was the man and woman I call my pastors. Tena and I served with them and under them for twelve years. I loved every second of the journey and would have been happy to remain there forever. But retirement came calling for them, and after a lifetime of pouring out, it was time to rest. I was a pace horse to my pastors and had no problem giving my robe, my tools, and my sword to their vision because I knew that their victories would be the victories I longed for myself.

Then there's David who had the unpleasant role as pace horse to an insecure Saul. The man he went to war for, built the kingdom with, and sang to when he was tormented was the same man who threw spears at him on multiple occasions. David gave Saul the same thing that Jonathan gave him. He could have killed him in a cave, but David took a piece of Saul's robe instead, showing him that he could have had your kingdom if he had wanted, but Saul chose to rip him out of his life because of his jealousy and fear just like this piece of robe. He declared Saul was his king and God's anointed. David would have served him to his dying breath if Saul had let him. David was Saul's pace horse.

I've served those same kinds of insecure and jealous leaders just like some of you have. All Saul ever accomplished by chasing David was to cause division and bring hurt and death upon the people. I ran as a pace horse to some of my pastors because I saw the faces of the people, even when they didn't or refused to see themselves. My heart ached each time God led us out because of the people. Spears have a way of making you move when they're being flung at you from the first chair. No one enjoys the reality of that type of hurt.

Our worship pastors just happen to be married to each other. The husband leads worship at the second campus with a dynamic team, and his wife leads at the main campus and is also the creative arts pastor. They both sit in a first-chair position for their department, but they download to their team and empower them greatly. He was once asked if I, as the pastor, was controlling and his reply was, "In the beginning, Pastor will walk with you hand-in-hand until you can stand alone. He will give you freedom as you earn it. When the time comes, he will get out of the way and let you do the job. Controlling? . . . No. Hands on? . . . Yes. But never forget the vision comes through him."

This is the fertile ground from which our church grows, and it's called healthy. Their vision for their departments is perfectly fitted with the vision that God has placed in me for the whole. They have removed their robes and weaponry and submitted them to the vision of the house. In return, they have created a healthy environment for growth.

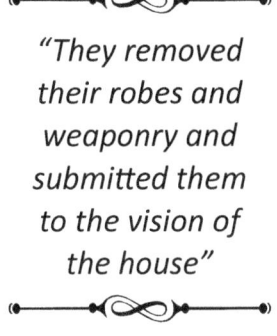

"They removed their robes and weaponry and submitted them to the vision of the house"

There's an elderly lady named Rachel at our church. She lives in a place of defeat all the time. She lost a daughter a few short years back and is constantly being beaten down by her husband at home. She would qualify to be a beaten horse as in chapter one. She will visit the church from time-to-time during the day, and no matter how hard we try to encourage her and lift her up, she just refuses to walk in victory. She sees the young people in our church and calls them pretty, when all she sees in herself is the opposite. Every now and then, our main campus worship pastor will disappear. You can see her work station shows that she's near, but we just can't find her. We will call and ask where she is, and she will say, "I just wanted to take Rachel to lunch and spend some time with her."

This is the spirit you either have or you don't. We can't create this heart for ministry in someone. She takes a few quality moments out of her super-busy schedule to lift an elderly lady's spirits. The powerful leader from the platform, beautiful and young, she takes time to see Rachel. Not just see as in an appointment like a doctor will see you now, she "sees" Rachel, and that's all that matters. Our worship pastors submitted their robes early on in our journey together. They possess the heart of the pace horse, and they both know the only way we're getting to the finish line is together.

Being more than a pace horse is not becoming rebellious to the one out front. Our worship pastors get it. Our campus pastor and team get it. Our children's leaders and youth teams get it. Our servant leaders from the pastoral staff all the way down get it. Submitting your robe and sword to the vision of the house is not being suppressed or robbed of personal vision. It's being more than a pace horse. When we run together, each one becomes more than pace horse; they become winners.

So you're the associate pastor; you are more than pace horse, my friend. And what about you? Yeah, sitting at your desk, reading this chapter. You're not just one of the musicians on the team or just the camera guy in the back. And you, reading this on your lunch break, you're not just a youth helper on the team whose only job is to get pizza. And you, you know who you are, serving at the coffee bar, making sure pots are filled and cups available. And there for a minute you thought I would slip by and miss you. You're the one who fills the sanctuary. You're there to worship. You don't really have a role or title. You're just known as a worshipper.

All of you are more than a pace horse, and without you we couldn't run. The race is always a tough one, and you are such an important part of the team because you push us forward. You run beside the visionary. You make us want to run harder, and you make us want to win. You help us see faces every morning when we wake up. Sure you have submitted your robe to the vision of the first chair, but many hands make light work, just like many robes cover the whole team. You are more than a pace horse; you're the team that creates wins. Every face that's envisioned by the leader is a life changed, and that encounter is made possible by you.

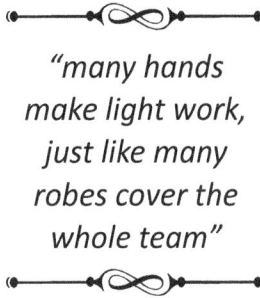

"many hands make light work, just like many robes cover the whole team"

Every fifth Sunday our church has a passion meeting. We schedule it for six p.m., and we use this time to give special attention to communion, baptisms, and intimate worship. During communion at one of these services, I looked back and saw a line of people all the way to the back of the sanctuary toward the rear doors. I couldn't help but allow my mind to drift back six years at a round table in the foyer with six people. We had launched back then with a vision of what we were seeing now. I went to three of those people and told them they were the reason for this many passionate people.

I told them in that first meeting that people would come, and they believed it. I knew God had placed that in my heart. I could see the people lined up in my mind. Even if they couldn't see it with their physical eyes, they still believed in the vision. They ran beside Tena and I like strong pace horses. They challenged us to run harder and with every hurdle and obstacle we faced, they kept pace. They stripped themselves of their robes and cast them with the vision. We ran together, and the longer the line becomes as we race from here, the harder we will run.

I have sat in the second chair many times and for many years. I served great leaders and some not so great or maybe not even a leader at all. Our pastors, whom we loved, built us up and taught us the value of running a race well. I was more than a pace horse to them; I was part of the team. I helped make the wins possible and took great honor in that. So run and run hard because you may not understand your worth now, but rest assured that Jesus does.

Chapter 11

THE STALLION/ THOROUGHBRED

Everyone wants to be the stallion. I'm pretty sure no one ever pictures themselves as a supporting character in their own story, so when we imagine our lives, I think it's just easier to see the stallion rather than the nag. The stallion is the destination; he's the top of the food chain of thoroughbreds. He just has it all together. His mane is braided and his tail combed. His coat glistens in the sunlight. He owns the ground he walks on with his command of attention and stately gate. He towers above the earth, hooves pounding. The earth trembles under his feet, and the thunder claps when he runs. The air flows through his nostrils like a wind tunnel. He owns the air he breathes and the soil he stands upon. This is the stallion; picture him as you wish because he's unaffected by the

> *"Everyone wants to be the stallion, but how many are willing to do what it takes to get there"*

thoughts and opinions of the crowd. Everyone wants to be the stallion, but how many are willing to do what it takes to get there.

Let me tell you about my friend. He's barely in his mid-twenties, and I dare to say he has preached over three thousand sermons. Drew grew up in the same small town I live in. His mother and father are some of our closest and dearest friends. You know, they're the ones you go on vacation with and turn around and schedule another trip because you enjoy their company so much. We've laughed and cried together so many times I can't count (most of those moments were spent laughing). We've closed down restaurants, cruise ships, and parking lots together with long hours of love and laughter. They are not just acquaintances, and Drew was not just one of those kids. He was—well—a stallion.

Everything seemed to always work well for Drew, and things fell into place for him seemingly very easily, not because he was lucky, but because he worked hard. Drew graduated into the youth group as he entered middle school. Tena and I were still youth pastoring at the time, and we quickly realized that he possessed a uniqueness about him as he turned from a little boy into a middle schooler. He would ask questions that I found myself having to study to find the answers for. I remember saying to Tena, "I believe this kid is being called to the ministry." Sure enough, a few weeks later, he called to let us know that he had heard from the Lord. God had made it very clear that he would be answering the call to ministry. He was barely a middle schooler. I asked him to take the pulpit in the youth room to speak, and he did so with confidence and poise. I made notes that night and later gave them to him as a gift. A few weeks later, I was asked to preach the main service for our pastor, and in secret Drew and I schemed a plan.

The Stallion/thoroughbred

We told no one. I would enter the pulpit, begin to preach, and simply walk off after a few minutes, and he would take over. We collaborated on the sermon topic, and I would start, and he would finish as the Holy Spirit directed each of us. That day came and still no one was privy to our plan. When I stepped away from the pulpit that night, the stallion stepped in, he spoke with anointing and maturity. Drew preached almost every night of his life all the way through middle and high school.

Most of those years, he had to be driven by his parents from church to church because he was not old enough to have a driver's license. They crisscrossed the southern states back and forth from town to town. They wore out tires and cars but kept moving forward. He preached in small churches, large churches, schools, tents, and every venue in between. Not only did he preach a sermon almost every night of his life through middle and high school, he also graduated valedictorian. At one time, he was the smartest kid I knew; now I think he's the smartest person I know. Drew never slowed down long enough to really be a teen, he quickly became college graduate Drew, then master's degree Drew, and soon we will call him Dr. Drew probably before he turns thirty.

He wasn't blessed because he was smart, nor were they wealthy. Being a stallion didn't get him to the top of the pecking order, either. He knows, and those of us around him know, that he is blessed because he was obedient to the call God had placed on his life. The Lord is the great orderer of our steps but it's our job to place our feet in the marks where his shoes

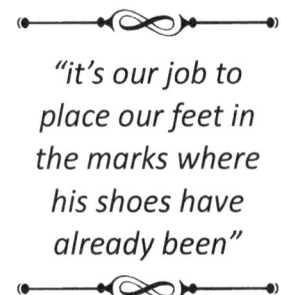

"it's our job to place our feet in the marks where his shoes have already been"

have already been. Drew chased after the right thing: that's the heart of the stallion.

Becoming the stallion doesn't reside in birthright or position. It doesn't matter if you are a workhorse, a stray, or a wild mustang; the key to becoming a stallion begins at the feet of Jesus. Stallions possess a certain bloodline that only comes through the shed blood of Jesus. All stallions have two things in common: they have Jesus's blood running through their veins, and they know how to use their platform. It doesn't matter what platform you began with, it only matters what platform you're standing on now. In real life, the stallion thoroughbred runs because that's the platform he's on. His job is to run his best race in the time he is given. After his racing career is over, his value remains high due to his stud service. His platform goes from all in, one hundred percent attention on training and racing to reproducing more race horses. Two platforms: one to produce, and the other to reproduce.

"It doesn't matter what platform you began with, it only matters what platform your're standing on now"

The Bible is filled with stories of Israel's many kings. Some of these kings produced with the platform they were given, but very few ever reproduced. Many used the platform given to them by God to orchestrate their evil will. They produced while in office but limited their production to exalt themselves. Some failed so miserably at reproduction that they killed their own offspring to protect their position. Jacob was not a king of Israel, but he was the leader of the family from whence the name *Israel* comes. He reproduced himself into the heads of the twelve tribes of Israel. His platform was the foundation that was laid to grow a family into a nation. God even produced in him a new name. On that platform he stood and reproduced and continues to reproduce through generations today.

David produced victories and reproduced warriors. He brought the people back to Jerusalem and used his platform to direct attention away from himself and onto God. He stood on the platform given to him and worshipped half naked in the streets in order to glorify his God. He reproduced not only kings but he also reproduced a passion and hunger for the Lord.

The opposite of David is a good example of a platform unwisely and selfishly used in a puppet king named Herod. He became so threatened by anyone and everyone, he chose to kill rather than reproduce. He added surrounding structures to the temple in Jerusalem until the temple of God became known as Herod's temple. He could have used his platform to glorify the Lord but chose it to glorify himself instead. He is known as Herod the Great, once again a failed platform opportunity wasted on pride and ego.

Men from a distant land we know as wise men traveled great distances to worship Jesus as the rightful king. They used their platform wonderfully. They set out on a journey through desert terrain and extreme conditions, and made themselves uncomfortable in the process to visit a newly born king they didn't know. They brought offerings, along with their worship. The offerings that God provided through them enabled the gospel to literally be moved into all the world. Those offerings quite possibly fed and housed the King of kings and his family throughout their early lives. What God gave through these men, Joseph was able to use as travel expenses to escape selfish King Herod's assassination orders.

Herod abused his platform. As a stallion, he had the chance to produce while he was in the race and to reproduce through

Jesus. Get hold of the enormity of the divine opportunity that Herod squandered. He was privileged to be in power during the time that Jesus was born. He had a platform that could have been used to elevate the name of Jesus and truly go down in history as Herod the Great. His platform could have been used to see wounds healed, sight restored to the blind, crippled bodies straightened, and sins forgiven. He missed out on every bit of that because he chose to hoard his platform for himself.

He used his platform to order a contract killing to be placed on the head of Jesus as a child, another opportunity squandered at the altar of pride and selfishness. The historian Josephus records that Herod became so depressed and miserable with his failing health that he attempted suicide to end his suffering. Even in his final days, he refused to use his platform to reproduce. Out of paranoia, he imprisoned his son. It is recorded that upon his failed attempt at ending his own life, the wailings from the palace were so loud that his son mistook that to mean his father had died. The son attempted to bribe the jailer to release him. That bribery was reported to Herod at which time he ordered his son to be executed. With only days left to live, Herod the "not so" Great devised a plan to have prominent leaders from every village in Judea imprisoned and ordered to be killed at the very moment of his death. His last act as king was to use his platform for death rather than reproduction. The plan however is reported to have never been carried out, but a life given by God had been wasted nonetheless.

What platform did you begin with? That doesn't have to be the platform to stand on now. My pastor is a wonderful example of a platform well used. He was a stallion that knew his retirement was soon, and yet he continued to reproduce. He was the district overseer for the denomination in our area.

He pastored the largest church in the district, but that's not what gave him his platform. He stood on a platform provided by Jesus, and he knew the value of reproduction. A young, aspiring minister approached him, seeking permission to plant a new church in his district and under his jurisdiction.

Now let me just add a note here that not only is church planting one of the core values of this denomination, it is also a dying outreach. I know this firsthand because I was one of those aspiring ministers who sought guidance and approval to start a new work. I was told by the powers that be not to get my hopes up because the district overseer would have to give his stamp of approval before the state office would give its blessings, and most pastors won't. A pastor who also acts as a district overseer that has a platform to reproduce and refuses—no way! You say, "There can't be a pastor who would refuse to see lives changed and sins forgiven." Oh, but yes way, there is, I'm afraid. I was the recipient of that rejection. Not one but two district overseers told me they didn't have the time or the desire to ordain such a church plant. Those pastors failed on their platforms.

It is not because I feel that I'm this great speaker or because I'm perfect. Our mission is to see people saved; simply put, that's job number one. Platforms are used for everything in this world. They are used for good and bad alike—for building up or for tearing down, for unity or for division, and for selfless acts or for selfish gain. But when we have the opportunity to use our platform to move the heart of Jesus to the world then there can be no greater accomplishment from any level. It is the pinnacle of the heart of the stallion.

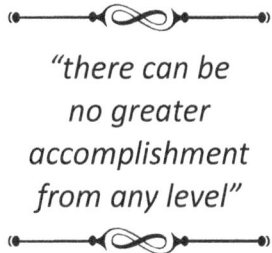
"there can be no greater accomplishment from any level"

Now you're probably wondering what happened to that young man and my pastor? This guy was just a kid. He and his equally young wife felt called to start a church. I'm not sure of his age, but I would guess when he approached my pastor with his vision for a church plant, he couldn't have been more than nineteen. Who gives a kid like that a chance to pastor a church and speak into the lives of people? My pastor took that chance. He helped that young man, encouraged him, gave him and his wife the chance of a lifetime, and they launched their little church on a stretch of road in the middle of nowhere with not much more than a family in attendance.

The young pastor continued to prove himself, and they stayed the course. They rented an old store on the weekends for quite some time until one day my pastor came calling. Another church on the district whose pastor was retiring would be needing a new leader. Their established church was only a few miles from this young man's new startup. They needed a new visionary and were close to maybe even having to close the doors and dissolve the church. My pastor could have used his platform to close that church and absorb that small congregation into our church, but instead he orchestrated the joining of the old church with the young pastor, and a marriage was born. They joined together, an older established congregation and a young visionary. Since that union, they have sold the old property, bought and built a new facility on the main highway, and continue to see lives changed and sins forgiven. My pastor used his platform to reproduce in another stallion and help him to create his own platform.

Paul has instructed us in his first letter to the Corinthian church to be a leader who uses the platform given to us wisely. In chapter eleven, he instructs, "follow me as I follow Christ." Be good stewards of the platform given by God. Make people want to follow you. Live and conduct your life on that platform in such a way that you can say as Paul has said, follow me and follow my platform because it is the same platform given to me by God. And when I stand on it, I will be pointing to my Savior. Paul didn't stand on a platform he created. He didn't stand on the platform that he began with, either.

He started out as different kind of stallion named Saul, but God had greater levels for him. Remember it's not the platform you started with that changes lives; it's the one God places you on that reproduces. If left to his own agenda, Saul the Pharisee would have gone down in history as one of the most ruthless and heartless terrorists of the Christian faith the world has ever known. He would have used his platform to produce pain and destruction. God elevated him to a new platform.

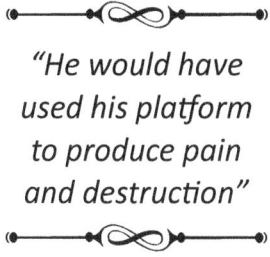

"He would have used his platform to produce pain and destruction"

God took this misguided Pharisee terrorist who had built his reputation on a lifeless platform and put in him the true heart of a stallion. Saul the Pharisee failed his platform, but Paul the apostle stood high on the stage that God anointed him with and reproduced life into churches, regions, and ministers. He produced life from a prison cell that continues to reproduce in our hearts today. We read, memorize, learn, and quote from the teachings and words that once were bound in the heart of the vilest and harshest of persecutors.

So what does your platform look like? Whatever platform you're on is the one you're advertising. People in the world today want Jesus; they just don't want the Jesus they're seeing. Maybe it's because for some, you've possessed the intentions of Paul, but you have Saul's actions. Take a look around and ask yourself, "Do I have what it takes to become a stallion?"

I'm going to answer that question with a question: What platform are you on now, and does it look like the platform you desire? You may not feel like you're stallion or thoroughbred material, but let me assure you that you are more than a pace horse, and stallion blood is just as available to you as it was to Paul the apostle.

The same blood that flowed through the heart of Billy Graham the evangelist is the same blood that can create your platform right now. Yes, the same pedigree that saw healing, salvation, and life can be yours for the asking. That ole mean Saul the persecutor wrote in his letter to the Roman church from his new stallion platform as Paul the servant of God: "that if we confess with our mouths that Jesus is Lord and believe in our hearts that God raised him from the dead then we shall be saved" (Romans 10:9–10). He also didn't fail to mention in verse 13 that "whosoever calls on the name of the Lord shall be saved."

Let me help you elevate your platform. Let me help you get the right blood applied to your life. Let me help you pray this simple prayer of salvation: "Lord, according to your Word, I repent of my sins, and I ask that your blood be applied to my life. I ask you to forgive me of my sins. I acknowledge you as Lord and Savior, and I thank you that I am the whosoever. In your name I pray, amen!" That scripture in Romans basically says to confess with our mouths and to mean what we say and as a result of that prayer we are changed and forgiven. If you prayed that prayer then congratulations, you've been elevated to thoroughbred status. Your old platform is gone. Use your new stallion platform wisely. Produce for Jesus, and reproduce through Jesus.

One final stallion I would like to mention is the one the conqueror rides into town on before going out to create great victories. You can find him in Matthew 21, tied to a post outside the house. But this stallion's not so easy to spot. He's possibly the only thing of value the owner possesses, and Jesus chooses him for his triumphant ride into Jerusalem the Sunday before his great victory. He's just an ordinary untamed donkey. An obscure little colt at daybreak would stand on a different platform midday. The ordinary that once was tethered to a post would become the centerpiece of extraordinary.

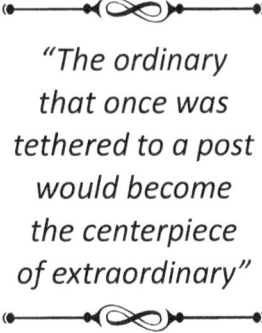

"The ordinary that once was tethered to a post would become the centerpiece of extraordinary"

A stallion that began as a donkey—who would have ever imagined that? He heard every hosanna and felt the wind from each waving palm branch as he passed by. He was more than a pace horse and more than a donkey; he was now a stallion, and he used his platform wisely. When all the noise had died down and the party was over, when the cleaning crews arrived and the people were silent, the little donkey went back home. He still looked like a donkey, his back still swayed, and his belly sagged. His stature remained petite and his ears still pointed. But his platform had been changed. The world may say that's not a stallion because stallions carry kings —yeah, that's what he did. Well, he can't qualify because that position is reserved for royalty— yeah, he carried the King over all kings. But you don't get what I'm saying, the party, the shouts, and palms are for stallions— yeah, exactly. You see, it doesn't matter what platform you started with; it only matters which one you're standing on now.

Chapter 12

THE STAMPEDE

There's a common thread that runs through the heartbeat of every horse. It's the one thing that connects and binds each one together, and that is they're all horses. It doesn't matter whether you think of yourself as the workhorse, the mare, or even the beaten horse; you're still a horse. Put them all together, and they form a stampede. No one notices if one is black and the other brown; all they see is the herd. The pack doesn't discriminate; it just runs, and it runs as a team. It accomplishes together what the individual can't.

A single horse in the open can barely be seen from long distances, but a stampede creates a presence. The ground shakes, and the sound of many hooves thunder across the landscape. The dust boils, and all eyes are drawn to the mob. There are beaten horses in that herd, running side-by-side with the stallion. Workhorses, mares, and strays keeping stride as they power

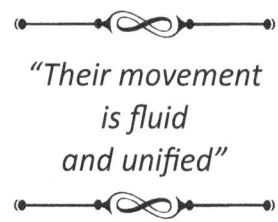

"Their movement is fluid and unified"

forward. They were built to run. They are all more than pace horses; they're one heartbeat. Their movement is fluid and unified.

The reason for writing this book is to reach out to the *one* and let you know that you are more than a pace horse. The same God who made you made all the others, past and present.

As I read and study the Bible, I find some interesting truths along this line of thinking. Take note that God has an order in which He operates. He seemed to always give dreams to the king but somehow gave the interpretation to the slave. He leveled the playing field by flowing through king and servant alike.

Joseph was in prison and locked away in an Egyptian jail, betrayed by his brothers, falsely accused by his owner's wife, and forgotten by society. Then God gave the king of Egypt a dream that he couldn't answer. Fortune tellers and magicians failed to appease the king's torment until a slave was brought in to save the day. Joseph interpreted Pharaoh's dream with pinpoint accuracy. God had given the slave kid the code to see what no other, not even the king, could envision. Joseph was more than a pace horse, whether his location was prison or palace. Joseph was promoted to the second chair that day. He was placed in leadership over his accusers, his former owner, and over the people. A king had locked arms with a slave—a stallion and beaten horse running side-by-side, a thoroughbred and lead pony stride for stride. They formed a union and saved a kingdom from famine and thousands of lives from certain death. I guess you could say God created a stampede with two horses to lead the way.

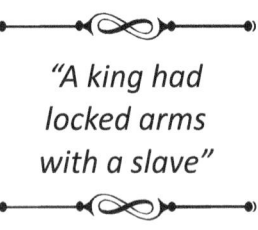
"A king had locked arms with a slave"

The Stampede

From my view there are two types of stampedes: the one coming in and the one going out. The one coming in is the larger of the two. It's the one that has the addict, school teacher, and alcoholic running side-by-side. These are the people who need the church more now than ever before. In that pack, we can find everyone from the suburban housewife and soccer mom to the overworked husband and father who has no time left for his kids. This stampede is full of the hurting and broken. Some are easy to spot, and others are just better at hiding it. They're coming, and they need a strong and powerful representation of Christ to speak life and healing into each one. They're coming with thunderous hooves and dust boiling into the air to mark their arrival.

The problem is the incoming stampede is much greater than the one going out. The church is sending out stampeders at an alarmingly slower rate than the world. While the church closes doors, the world is creating greater stampedes by the second. Jesus gave us ample warning in the book of Luke, chapter 10, when He stated that the harvest is plenty, but the laborers are few. In verse 1, He sent stampedes out before Him. They were sent out into the towns but were instructed to stay in people's homes where they were accepted. He instructed them to eat and stay with the homeowners. Sitting for a meal with someone is one of the most intimate things we can do with another. When you share a meal, you learn their heart. Learn their heart and win the family. Win the family and win the town. Jesus knows what He's doing.

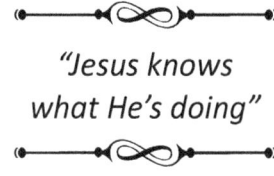

"Jesus knows what He's doing"

There's a great harvest happening all around us. God has called us out and sent us to reach the towns and cities. That's where the harvest is plentiful. He has given us the recipe for the proper stampede into each of these communities, and that is to reach the "one." Reach the *one*, and the city will eventually fall.

I took a trip to visit my dear friends one day. They have always been close to us much like family. The wife was friends with my sister in school, and we spent many days serving together in our church. I had heard they were out of church, so we loaded up like a stampede to their house. Their home was a staging point for ATV rides, and on that day there was several others there. I talked with my friends and invited them to church, but one family member was there that I had only met maybe once. Jason is his name, and we were cordial and spoke briefly.

Jason later started attending our church with his wife and son. That one brief encounter between the ATV trailer and a tree opened a door for Jason to enter. He and his wife came to church, but it didn't stop there. He invited his mother who had prayed for years that her family would come to Christ. But wait there's more: he brought his brother and his family, and not too many Sundays ago, Jason's mother held her granddaughter in her arms at the altar as she gave her heart to the Lord. I looked into the eyes of that grandmother in the floor with her adult granddaughter wrapped tightly and said to her, "One at a time, my friend, one at a time."

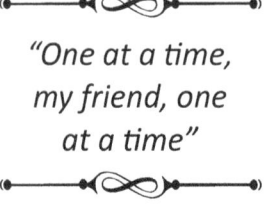

"One at a time, my friend, one at a time"

This grandmother prayed for this day since she was only a mother. She had dreamed of the day she would stand side-by-side with her family in worship. On Mother's Day, not only was her row full, but so was her heart. Jason now plays electric guitar on the worship team, his wife Sarah is the high school youth pastor, and his mother serves in hospitality. They are as much my family as anyone could be. Learn the heart and win the family; win the family and win the town. That's what a stampede looks like.

The world doesn't need more stampeders, but the church does because the harvest is great but not so much for the laborers. They may not look like you think and may not even be easy to spot. You may have to look over by the truck, somewhere between the trailer and a shade tree. You may be one of them right now, and you're thinking I can't be a harvester and join a stampede for Jesus. That's exactly what I said several years ago. Then I switched teams.

I've walked in the hoofmarks of each of these horses. I know what it feels like to run alone and to run with the herd. I've wanted to quit on several occasions. I've asked God to put me to work, and I've asked Him to fire me. I've asked Him, "Why me?" more times than I can count. Why me to be persecuted and why me to lead. I've asked him what I did wrong and what I did right. I learned lessons the easy way and mostly the hard way. I've wondered what He saw in me that I and everyone else couldn't. But He chose me a dyslexic, ADHD ditchdigger with a southern drawl and confusing speech. He chose me just like He has chosen you. It doesn't matter what label you have worn in the past or maybe are wearing right now. Labels have a way of falling to the ground around Jesus. Take it from me—if He wants me in the stampede, then rest assured, He wants you. You're worth more than you think. Your value doesn't reside on old platforms. Your value is in Christ and Him alone.

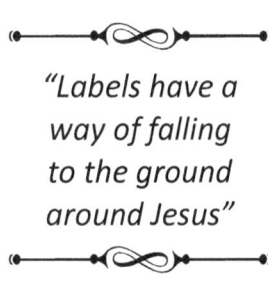

"Labels have a way of falling to the ground around Jesus"

Remember this one last thought after you have read this and still feel like disqualifying yourself from the stampede, God used murderers as deliverers, adulterers to be kings, dreamers to save nations, donkeys for triumph, and fishermen to change the world. And if He can turn ditchdiggers into pastors, then he can use you. Welcome home.

CPSIA information can be obtained
at www.ICGtesting.com
Printed in the USA
LVHW011408220819
628496LV00004B/5/P